Nature's Secrets
in

Health &
Vitality

D0317984

A Complete Guide to

Natural Health
Nutritional Supplements
and
Herbal Remedies

Brendan Salmon

B. A. (Hons)

ISBN 1 870703 17 0

To Mum and Dad who have been the main inspiration behind the writing of this book and whose efforts and strength of character have made everything possible. Also to Dolly whose sense of humour and home cooking have been a revelation throughout.

First Imprint, Vitapress 1991
Second Imprint Francis Joseph 1995

© Brendan Salmon 1995

Typesetting Francis Salmon
Cover Evelene Blanche Gregory
Line Drawings Peter McGaffin

Printed and bound in the United Kingdom
Francis Joseph London
ISBN 1 870703 17 0

Preface

Health is a subject which rightly pre-occupies many of us and which presently receives vast media attention, from newspapers, radio and television. There is little doubt that most people are generally confused as to what exactly alternative medicine stands for, about which foods form a healthy diet, which supplements or medicines one ought to use, whether to visit the doctor, homeopath, chemist or health shop. It is hardly surprising that confusion reigns supreme when the media presents often erroneous information on natural medicine and appears to understand so little about the subject. Furthermore, there is no end to the number of health product companies exhorting the public to buy the answer to all their problems with promises of health, beauty, vitality and long-life. Just what is the public to do when confronted by teeming shelves of invitingly packaged and forcefully advertised health and beauty aids? It isn't surprising that people are somewhat bemused by it all.

This book is a simple effort to clarify some of the issues involved and to help bring the individual to a greater understanding of the philosophy of 'natural' or 'alternative' medicine and of the role of diet and lifestyle in health and disease.

Warning

All efforts to combat disease, illness or injury must be approved by a medical practitioner. No course of treatment should be undertaken without your doctor's consent. No liablility can be accepted by either publisher or author for errors, omissions or directives contained in this book.

CONTENTS

**Glossary Of Nutritional Supplements

*Common Ailments and their Natural Treatments

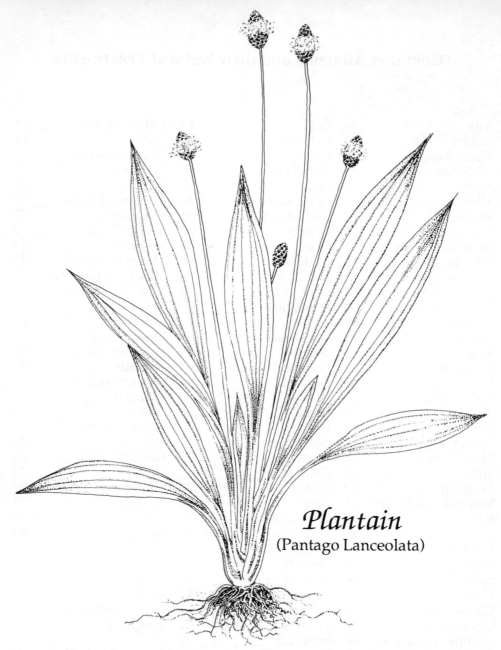

Plantain
(Pantago Lanceolata)

'Through the centuries healing has been practised by folk-healers who are guided by traditional wisdom that sees illness as a disorder of the whole person ... I would suggest that the whole imposing edifice of modern medicine, for all its breathtaking successes is ... slightly off balance ... The health of human beings is so often determined by their behaviour, their food and the nature of their environment...'
HRH Prince Charles at the 150th anniversary of the BMA

CHAPTER ONE

The Eight Healing Forces of Nature

One of the earliest pioneers of nature-cure medicine was Dr Bircher Benner who wrote *The Cure of Incurable Diseases*. In it he explained how a raw food dietary regime, consisting of fruits, vegetables, nuts, seeds, beans and cereal grains not only maintained vigorous health but was capable of arresting the progress of incurable diseases. He concluded that animal foods were deleterious to health and that raw plant foods contained living elements and energies which promoted positive wellbeing. He believed that nature-cure would one day become the major approach to the eradication of disease. Dr Bircher Benner was extra-ordinarily successful as a practitioner in his Austrian clinic and was a pioneer of the nature-cure movement.

The same conclusion was drawn from a totally unrelated study of a remarkable race of people who, up to the 1920's when they were first discovered, had been untouched by civilization. Since they exist in harmony with mother nature and as a consequence enjoy glorious good health, their story is worth pursuing.

The Hunzas live in a virtually inaccessible mountainous region between Afghanistan and India and as such had never come into contact with western civilization until their discovery in the 1920's. Such was the interest in this race of people that a British doctor, Sir Robert McCarrison, took it upon himself to make the hazardous journey to Hunza in order to monitor their health and lifestyle and to see if any lessons could be learned in the fight against disease in the western world. Many of his findings were published in UK medical journals but they appear to have been largely ignored over the last sixty years in favour of orthodox medicine. Sir Robert's writings expressed the view that the Hunzas were the finest specimens of human health imaginable, that disease was unknown, and that he never discovered one case of major illness in the period of time he spent there. Life expectancy could reach 140 years and their vitality and youthfulness was maintained well beyond 'normal' old age. Clearly it was important to study the lifestyle of the Hunzas. If such a disease-free existence could be maintained by these people, with all the related happiness which they apparently enjoyed, then surely it would be possible to take advantage of these findings and confront the problems of our own disease-ridden society.

The lifestyle of the Hunza is a simple one. They work ten hours each day on the land, sleep eight hours, pray, and maintain a very relaxed and unhurried approach to life. The air they breathe is crisp and fresh, the water is pure and sparkling and their food natural and organically grown.

Their diet is of particular interest as it does not contain any animal food. It consists of raw fruits, (in particular peaches and apricots), raw vegetables, all kinds of nuts and seeds, and cereal grains from which they make their own flour and bread. They frequently remove the kernel from apricots, from which they extract oil, using it as food and to oil their skin and hair. It has recently been discovered that apricot kernel seeds contain vitamin B17, otherwise known as Laetrile, which is believed to exert a significant anti-cancer action. The only animal food used by the Hunzas is small quantities of goat's milk which is consumed rarely and only on special occasions. It must also be mentioned that for several months of the year food is very sparse in Hunza and the community lives almost entirely without sustenance throughout this period, providing them with the opportunity to rid their bodies of toxins. This process will be explained more fully when the philosophy of nature-cure is considered.

As further proof of the dynamic relationship between diet and disease, experiments were set up by Sir Robert McCarrison with interesting but hardly surprising results. Experimental rats were used, as their choice of food resembles our own, and they were split into two groups. One group was given a Hunza diet of raw carrots, fruit, cereal, grains etc, and thrived, living to 120 years in human terms. Autopsies revealed no traces of disease. The other group was fed on a typical western diet of potatoes, white bread, butter and meat. These animals developed cancer and heart disease at an early stage, they aged prematurely and tended to be extremely violent. When this group were switched to the Hunza diet their disease conditions disappeared and their health was regained.

A question clearly needs answering. Where has this type of information and research disappeared to in the period since the 1920's? If a race of people are capable of maintaining perfect health through existing in harmony with the laws of nature, then it is clear that health only breaks down when these laws are infringed. Over the last few decades modern medicine has often ignored the relationship between environment and health and has frequently scoffed at the notion that diet may have a serious impact on the condition of human health. It has preferred, instead, to issue vast quantities of pharmaceutical medicines to a trusting and willing population, completely ignoring the underlying environmental causes of disease. This practice has generated enormous wealth but has undermined the physical and spiritual health of the nation, imposing on its people an incalculable degree of human suffering. The prescribing of medicines is clearly more lucrative than health education.

It is difficult though to blame doctors for this state of affairs considering that their medical education over the past few decades has been almost totally devoid of any emphasis on the science of nutrition. There has been little study of the consequence of environmental factors and diet on human health. Medical training is very obviously prescription orientated, favouring pharmaceutical medicines to the more wholesome herbal, homeopathic and nutritional remedies that are available. Through this lack of emphasis in training, doctors themselves are done a great disservice.

There are however many positive elements in modern medicine. Medical treatments in accidents and emergencies are indispensable and many serious disorders beyond the body's recuperative powers depend upon medicines to control their symptoms and pain. Surgery is essential in many circumstances, often relieving life-threatening conditions and allowing the body's recuperative powers to be liberated. It must be said that any treatment, whether it be open heart surgery, organ transplants or the use of antibiotics or pain killers can be nothing but commendable if it improves the quality of an individual's life.

There is little more likely to stir the emotions and induce a sense of pride than in caring for the health of those in need. The modern health service succeeds in this and doctors and nurses make stirling efforts for their patients. However, in spite of their successes, one must not be blinded to the fact that in the treatment of disease, orthodox medical philosophy has no proper concept of the dynamic relationship between man and his environment. As such they tend to treat diseases in a particular, narrow-sighted way. Whilst orthodox medicine concentrates on the disease, and frequently only on the symptoms, alternative medicine concerns itself more greatly with the mind, body and spirit; the cause of disease and its removal from the patient's environment and lifestyle.

Given the prejudiced slant of orthodox medical philosophy and training therefore, it is difficult to see how an orthodox medical practitioner can be in the best position to determine what is best for the individual patient. Many doctors have rejected the teachings of their medical training and have become more involved with the philosophy of alternative medicine. One such practitioner was Dr Richard McKarness who concentrated his energies on determining the effects of the environment on human health. He demonstrated that groups of patients suffering from a wide range of mental and physical disorders, when isolated in a chemically clean environment and fed solely on spring water often experienced complete relief from their ailments. He concluded thst the illnesses of his patients were often triggered by a sensitivity to air (petro-chemicals), impure food, additives, chemical sprays or a particular food allergy. Ailments such as eczema, depression, schizophrenia, lethargy, bowel disorders, migraines, and many more, were all treated successfully by Dr McKarness using his methods. He left the country several years ago for Australia due to lack of financial support from the medical authorities and what he described as the envy, apathy and disinterest of his fellow doctors.

The Philosophy Of Natural Medicine

The philosophy of natural medicine, or nature-cure, is based around the premise that the health of a living organism is maintained by the elements of air, water and sunshine and by observance of the eight healing forces of nature, and also that the human organism contains within it, as part of its life force, a miraculous power for self-healing. This can be readily witnessed in the healing of broken bones, the healing of wounds and the body's ability to recover from illness and disease. If allowed to flourish in a natural environment in harmony with the laws of nature then good health will be bestowed upon all living things. The central core of the philosophy of natural medicine is that health can be maintained or re-built only through observance of the eight healing forces of nature. These are:

1   Air
2   Water
3   Exercise
4   Sunshine and Light
5   Fasting
6   Sleep and Rest
7   Positivity
8   Food

Air

Provides oxygen which is transported through the bloodstream by haemoglobin. Man cannot survive longer than a few minutes without air so its importance is self-evident. Fresh outdoor air contains negative ions which induce well-being and vitality. Positive ions which accumulate indoors and in built-up areas have the opposite action and tend to induce lethargy and fatigue. Fresh air is a potent rejuvenating force and a therapeutic tonic to the whole system. There are few people whose spirit and constitution are not invigorated by oxygenation of the bloodstream through outdoor pursuits in fresh, unpolluted air.

Exercise

Exercise is essential in activating the body's rhythms. It oxygenates the blood stream and maintains the health of the internl organs and muscles. It stimulates the circulatory system and the proper functioning of the heart and engenders health and vitality. For the person who is out of condition, exercise ought to be taken gradually, as a vigorous work-out on a deconditioned system appears to absorb inordinate quantities of vitality. It is thus essential to acclimatise gradually. The major cause of premature death in western society relates to diseases of the circulatory system, in particular heart disease, strokes and hardening of the arteries. The antidote to this epidemic of circulatory diseases will clearly implicate diet and exercise as the major therapeutic agents. Exercise also increases the body's metabolic rate and is thus invaluable for those who are overweight.

Water

Water is essential to all bodily functions and to life itself. It is taken internally either directly or indirectly through fruits and vegetables. Tap water is quite often undesirable due to toxic elements that it may contain - such as lead, copper, aluminium, nitrates, etc. Bottled spring water is a healthy alternative and water filters are available which remove many of the harmful elements found in tap water. It is not recommended to drink large quantities of water, thirst alone should dictate the amount consumed. Water is also used externally in alternative medicine in treatments which include cold compresses, salt baths, saunas and use of swimming pools.

Sunshine and Light

It goes without saying that the sun is the source of all life on this planet, but it is important in certain less obvious ways. Light stimulates photo-receptors at the back of the human eye which in turn stimulate the bodies hormonal secretions. People who rarely come into contact with daylight are likely to experience impaired well-being and vitality. People who are removed from light altogether for long periods experience severe damage to their health. Sunshine also creates vitamin D in our bodies through the action of sunlight on the oils of our skin. Unfortunately, due to the habit of wearing clothes and washing off skin oils with soap, not to mention the lack of sunshine in our climate, vitamin D requirements are often not met. The healing force of sunshine combines particularly well with the therapeutic action of air and exercise, all three being satisfied by outdoor pursuits.

Fasting

This requires abstention from food in order to liberate the body's own healing powers. This particular healing force is often used in nature-cure clinics with outstanding success but it ought to be attempted under medical supervision only. It would not be advisable to attempt to fast at home surrounded by the hustle and bustle of the modern world, though short periods on fruit alone would be quite safe. I have personally witnessed many examples of the miraculous healing powers of fasting and I would like to mention one in particular. The case involves a young man of 24 years named Julian who was suffering from the debilitating consequences of ulcerative-colitis. He weighed approximately 6.5 stones (90 lbs), his back was bent in a severe stoop and he could walk only in a painful shuffle. He was pitifully unwell and his face was gaunt and etched with pain. He had been under medical supervision for six years without any success, indeed he had deteriorated steadily over this period. For the first month of his treatment at Tyringham Naturopathic Clinic, England, Julian was fed purely on fruit and vegetable juice in order that the body's self healing mechanism be released and to initiate the necessary detoxification from the medicines he had been using. During this period he studied the philosophy of nature-cure and slowly came to learn that his health was in his own hands and that his own body could heal itself. I can only say that when Julian left the clinic he was a different person from the one who had arrived. His stoop had gone, he bounced jauntily around and wore a huge smile. Nobody healed Julian, he had healed himself. His body had contained the power to heal his disease. Furthermore, Julian had understood the power of nature and his destiny was now in his own hands.

Sleep and Rest

Sleep and rest are the healing forces which recharge the system and renew the life-force. In the threat of disease or illness, sleep and rest are the main therapeutic agents, liberating the body's own healing powers. Persons suffering from sleep deprivation are likely to seriously impair their health and their ability to cope with life. Clearly the best time for sleep is night-time as the body's twenty-four hour clock has been set over a period of millions of years of evolution. People who work at night often find day-time sleep unsatisfying and incomplete and are more prone to ill-health, fatigue and nervous complaints. Animals catnap throughout the day whenever fatigue ensues and this is a technique mastered by some people with positive benefits. Sleep is more complete and rejuvenating on an empty stomach as the body is liberated from any pre-occupation with the digestion of food.

Positivity

Just as positive health induces a sense of positive thought and wellbeing, the converse is also true. A positive and cheerful disposition will exert a profound and definite influence upon the secretions and workings of the human system. It is true to say that many diseases, including cancer, are likely to occur after periods of stress and trauma and, whilst it is impossible to remove emotional pain from the human condition, it may be possible to avoid the onset of illness through positive thought and the development of a positive personal philosophy to life. It must be said here that a prerequisite to sound mental health is vigorous physical health and this is a goal to be pursued through observance of the physical laws of nature.

The will to live is a significant influence over our life chances and thus a general attitute of positive thought will keep illnesses at bay and increase our life span. Perhaps it would be worthwhile to liberate a degree of positive thought and reflect from time to time on morale raising aspects of the human condition whether it be heroism, compassion or the dawn of consciousness.

In consideration of consciousness, it might be described as a higher form of enlightenment which counters the more primitive passions of ego, vanity and self-interest and enables the individual to experience an empathy with the world around him, a tolerance and compassion toward his fellow man.

The individual can do no greater service to himself and to humanity than to ally himself with the forces of higher consciousness whether it be through personal development or through active participation in humanitarian issues. It is certain that the healing force of positive thought is an untapped source of human joy and no matter what the individual's personal circumstances are, there are few situations which do not benefit from the gift of hope and the power of positivity. The pursuit of happiness in which we all take part is ultimately a pursuit of spiritual joy and in this scenario we play a leading role. Through meditation, introspection or thought development it is possible to dissipate some of the tensions of everyday life and to develop the gift of gratitude for the positive elements each day contains. Modern day materialism, with its relentless pursuit of money, possessions and superficial pleasures does not seem particularly conducive to human happiness. Higher considerations of inner development and inner peace and mastery of the art of positive dynamism are more likely to be conducive to true happiness.

Food

Such is the importance of this healing force, that it is dealt with fully in the next chapter.

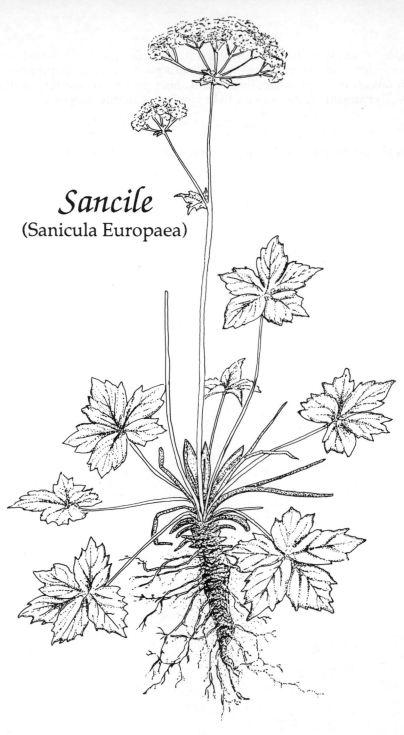

Sancile
(Sanicula Europaea)

CHAPTER TWO

Food for Health

During his evolutionary development over millions of years in the rain forests of the African continent, man has evolved with a physical requirement for food of plant origin, not animal origin. Much is made of the image of pre-historic man using guile and expertise to kill animals for food, but while there may be some element of truth in this contention, it is clear that the mastery of fire was necessary to convert raw flesh foods into something more palatable. One can say without fear of contradiction that there are not too many humans, either in the present day or in the misty pasts of history, who would be prepared to kill an animal and consume its raw flesh at the moment of death as would any meat-eating predator. That this idea of consuming raw flesh is so repellant to most of us is a clear indication that man is not naturally carnivorous. The mastery of fire to disguise the taste and texture of raw meat was clearly a pressing necessity and indeed it was in mastering fire that man showed the creativity and intelligence which millions of years of evolution had shaped him for - and all on a plant food diet!

Adapted to meat?

The switch to a partial meat-eating regime requires a different digestive apparatus than the consumption of plant foods and in the process of adaptation to this new food, we have placed an enormous physiological stress on the human organism.

Meat eaters manifest in general a much higher predisposition towards various illnesses and diseases than do vegetarians. Clearly man has had only limited success in the process of adaptation to flesh foods. It must be remembered that animals adapt and evolve around their particular environments. The giant ant-eater, for example, developed an extremely long snout in order that it could bury deep into ants nests for food. Lions, tigers and other carnivorous animals are all perfectly adapted to hunting and killing for food.

It is clear that food, its constant accessibility and ingestion is a major formative element in the development of any species. Man has adapted to and evolved around a plant food diet of fruits, vegetables, nuts, seeds and beans and it is in consequence these foods which ought to form the main bulk of his diet in the pursuit of maximum health and vitality. A return to a raw plant food diet would remove many of the major diseases of civilization and would alleviate untold pain and suffering throughout the human race.

Flesh foods, namely meat and fish, are not foods which one would be inclined to eat raw. This is a good indication that they are not particularly well suited to human consumption and digestion. They may be particularly suited to a carnivorous predator but manifestly not to herbivorous man. Flesh foods do provide high concentrations of protein but as this is not in short supply, even in a strictly plant food diet, then it becomes an expensive luxury. Further, all animal flesh contains purine bodies and animal fats which generate high levels of toxic by-products when digested in the system. These toxins and fats then circulate freely in the bloodstream and sow the seeds for arterial damage, circulatory troubles and heart disease. Even fish, currently promoted as a healthy food is still dead flesh, generating high levels of waste poisons in the bloodstream in the process of digestion. Fish also has the disadvantage of being taken from heavily polluted seas, whether the contamination be toxic by-products from industry, sewage, or nuclear wastes.

The heavy consumption of meat and its by-products is a more serious cause for concern due to its implication in many major diseases. First and foremost amongst these are heart and circulatory troubles. An article in an American medical journal in 1969 commented:

'American men killed in the Korean war showed, even at the age of twenty two, striking signs of arteriosclerotic disease (furring of the arteries) as compared with Korean soldiers who were free of this damage to their blood vessels. The Americans were well fed with plenty of milk, butter, eggs and meat. The Koreans were basically vegetarians'.

There is conclusive evidence that a diet high in saturated fats (animal fats) leaves plaque residues on the artery walls causing hardening of the arteries, this being a major cause of heart disease and strokes. One half of all deaths in the United States is believed to be caused by arterial disease, making it one of the major killers in man's history. Meat eating is also linked to that other great killer in western society, cancer. Laboratory animals are often doctored with medications that check disease and improve output, but the result is that animals' flesh frequently contains penicillin, arsenic, female hormones or diethylstilboesterol, all known to produce cancer. Meat often contains pathogenic bacteria and is responsible for four out of five cases of food poisoning in Great Britain. Meat is also implicated in constipation, appendicitis and cancer of the bowel, principally due to its lack of fibre. Dietary roughage encourages the passage of food and waste products through the system and maintains a healthy bacterial flora. Meat, due to its difficulty of digestion, often decomposes and putrefies in the human gut, releasing poisonous toxins into the bloodstream which have an adverse effect on mind and body. On moral grounds one may condemn meat-eating on the basis that it creates a demand for the slaughter of sentient, docile animals. However, this is not the only moral reason for shunning meat-eating, for animal proteins are an extravagant luxury in a world where the majority of people are short of decent food. Animals consume twenty pounds of plant food protein to provide one pound of animal protein. It could be that, if the land where cattle graze were turned over to the production of plant proteins, then a large step forward could be taken in solving the world's food shortages. In order that the affluent minority of the west can indulge themselves in an extravagant yet unnecessary luxury, crops that could help solve the world's food shortages are fed to cattle, to yield a small return in protein. Ironically, the grain to feed these cattle is often imported from starving nations instead of being used to feed the hungry people who produce it.

Adapted to dairy products?

With regards to dairy products man is the only animal to consume the milk of another animal after being weaned from mother's milk. As a consequence to this infringement of the law of nature, large sections of the population are predisposed towards heart disease, arterial damage and other circulatory disorders related to the excessive use of milk and its high concentrations of unsaturated fat. Cows' milk fed to babies is a particularly unwise habit. It contains twice as much protein as mothers' milk creating difficulties of digestion and is intended for the rapid development of a calf rather than the slower development of a small human. Cows' milk also lacks the right composition of nutrients and antibodies which are essential to the development of the child's immune system. Cows' milk is further implicated in the development of allergies, infantile eczema and various digestive troubles. As pointed out earlier, man is the only animal that consumes milk after being weaned. Clearly milk and its derivatives of butter, cream and cheese are enjoyable foods and this alone may account for its wholesale popularity. However, when one considers the slick advertising of milk as a 'natural', wholesome food containing protein and essential minerals, one may recognise that a degree of conditioning invokes excessive consumption. Not too many people would be inclined towards pigs' milk, sheep's milk or even mother's milk and, if commonsense prevails, it must be admitted that cows' milk is neither a wholesome or natural food for human consumption. This is borne out by scientific research, which having revealed the injurious action of animal fats through much pain staking research and expense, merely confirms the self-evident.

Milk then, and its by products ought to be used sparingly as a concession to enjoyment rather than to necessity, preferring the low fat products of cottage cheese, yoghurt and low fat milk. These foods contain protein, essential vitamins and minerals and do, it must be conceded, lend themselves to the improvement of many culinary dishes.

Food allergies

Cereal grains (particularly wheat, oats, and barley) are highly nutritious foods containing many carbohydrates for energy and much fibre. It is, however, unlikely that they have played a large part in man's early evolution and as such they can cause problems. Wheat, in particular, is a relatively recent addition to man's diet having only been consumed over the last several thousand years when man began to farm the soil. In terms of evolution this is a very short time and as such man is not particularly well adapted to it. Whilst most people can consume this food in quantity without any ill effect, some find that they are allergic to it. Wheat is the number one allergen in our modern diet, more people being made ill by this food both mentally and physically than by any other. The principle reason for this appears to be a high gluten content which is badly tolerated by many people. If you feel unwell and cannot find a solution it may be wise to cut this food, and all its white flour derivatives, out of your diet and monitor the results. Problems with gluten can range from headaches to lethargy to bowel disturbances, and many other varied complaints. For those able to tolerate gluten, wheat, oats, barley and other cereal grains can be consumed liberally, for they are highly nutritious.

Dairy products are another major allergen in the modern diet, and are also a very recent addition to man's diet. The same applies to dairy products as to cereal grains. If you feel persistently unwell without cause, then it maybe worth while omitting this group of foods from your diet for a short while and observing the results. Cow's milk can be substituted with goat's milk which is easier to digest and is considered superior in its nutritional composition.

Eggs also fall into this category, being a modern food and needing heat to disguise the unpalatability of their raw state. They are one of five major allergens (the other four being cereals, dairy products, tea and coffee) and should be watched carefully by those suffering from food sensitivities. For those tolerant of eggs, one or two weekly should do no harm to one's health, preferring free range eggs to those from factory farms.

Virtues of a natural diet

It is clear then that a natural diet for man, on the evidence of both commonsense and scientific research, should comprise principally of plant foods; fruits, vegetables, nuts, seeds, beans and cereal grains. Some concession can be made to the use of low fat dairy products, though animal flesh foods are fairly indefensible on both moral and health grounds. If they are to be used in one's diet, then low fat varieties are preferable such as chicken, fowl and fish, but should be used in strict moderation.

The idea that animal protein foods are needed for strength and stamina is a fallacy, the converse is actually true. Maximum strength and vitality is experienced on a diet high high in natural carbohydrate and low in proteins. Countless scientific studies have been undertaken which show that well-being, stamina and endurance increase markedly on a low protein diet and particularly when the proteins are obtained from plant foods. This should not be too surprising as the healthiest tribes and races on the planet eat little if any animal foods. For anyone still dubious about whether a vegetarian diet will support their strength, Thomas Paar, the most long lived man in British history, was born in 1483 died in 1635 and stayed physically active until his death at the age of 152. He was a vegetarian.

A natural diet comprises of 70% fruits and vegetables and 30% small quantities of the other more concentrated foods (protein, carbohydrates and fats of plant origin). This dietary regime will maintain a pure, alkaline, well nourished blood stream containing all the necessary elements for energy and repair.

The myth that large quantities of animal proteins are required to maintain health has no doubt been perpetrated by the vested interests of the food industry. A look at the facts does not support this contention however. Foods at one time were classified as first class proteins, comprising mainly animal foods and second class proteins usually consisting of plant foods. This classification is now totally discredited with all the amino acids essential for body repair and general health being provided adequately by a mixed diet of plant foods. For example, nuts and seeds if combined with cereal grains, as in a muesli breakfast, provide a complete range of amino acids and proteins without the saturated fat and lack of fibre which characterises animal foods. Besides this the protein content of nuts and beans compares favourably with those of animal foods. An analysis of beef-steak for

18

example shows it contains 29 grams of protein, 242 calories, 14 grams of animal fat and negligible amounts of nutrients. Almonds however per 100 grams contain 20% protein, 580 calories, large quantities of unsaturated fatty acids and a high proportion of calcium. Soya beans contain 40 grams of protein per 100 grams of weight with 23 grams of unsaturated fatty acids and large proportions of vitamins, trace elements and amino acids. Protein occurs in most plant foods, particularly in nuts, seeds, beans, wheat-germ, cereal grains, lentils, peas and brewers yeast. Fruits, dried fruits and vegetables also contain some protein though in smaller quantities. It would be exceedingly difficult, if not impossible, for anyone consuming a diet of natural plant foods to become protein deficient. When one considers the possible inclusion of dairy products in the diet, the problem is more likely to be one of too much protein, rather than too little.

Veganism

Veganism (the abstention from all foods of animal origin including dairy products), provides all the elements and nutrients necessary to maintain vigorous health and vitality. It is highly likely that vegans, living exclusively on plant foods and avoiding all the refined and processed foods of modern society, will attain the highest possible degree of health and the greatest insurance against the major diseases of civilization. It has been suggested that one nutrient which may be lacking in the vegan diet is vitamin B12. Deficiencies do occur though they are more prevalent amongst meat-eaters than vegans. Whilst it appears that most vegans do not show any symptoms of vitamin B12 deficiency, either because sufficient is obtained from plant foods (brewers yeast is the best source) or because the body is capable of synthesising its own, it may be wise to take a vitamin B12 supplement to assuage any shock to the system which may be experienced when switching from a diet high in animal foods to a vegan diet of plant foods.

Veganism is certainly more morally justifiable than vegetarianism, as it does not necessitate the activities of the dairy industry in producing milk. Even this seemingly innocent activity creates hardship, as cows are kept in a constant state of pregnancy to provide milk and are separated from their calves immediately after birth so that milk can be sold, an action that produces much distress for both mother and calf. In the case of veal production, the calves are then either slaughtered immediately or isolated in crates for many weeks, sustained by an iron deficient diet which produces the white meat demanded by the public.

Veganism is the acid test of humanitarianism and compassion and will surely develop greater credibility and a larger number of devotees as time passes and man's consciousness increases.

Saturated and unsaturated fats

At this point we must consider the role of fats in the diet. Animal fats (saturated) are clearly injurious to health and should be avoided. Fats or oils of plant food origin (unsaturated) are essential to health and cannot be omitted from the diet without ill-health ensuing. These unsaturated fatty acids or essential fatty acids are found in nuts, seeds, beans and cereal grains such as walnuts, peanuts, cashew nuts, almonds, soya beans, sunflower seeds, olives and wheatgerm etc. A diet containing these foods will ensure a complete intake of the essential fatty acids required for health. The oils extracted from them are frequently used in cooking although it should be borne in mind that heat destroys the properties of plant oils and should be used only sparingly if at all as a culinary aid.

Any oil used in salad dressings (e.g Olive oil and Sunflower oil), or taken from the spoon to correct a dietary deficiency, should be cold-pressed which indicates that the oil has been expressed with pressure rather than with heat. This preserves its nutritional composition. A deficiency of essential fatty acids can cause skin complaints including dry scaly skin, dermatitis and eczema. These fatty acids are also used in the treatment of pre-menstrual tension, being a precursor of hormones called prostaglandins, in multiple sclerosis due to their importance in maintaining the health of the myelin sheath around the nerves and in prevention of thrombosis due to their ability to reduce high blood cholesterol levels. Oil of Evening Primrose is a particularly well known source of essential fatty acids due to its high level of linoleic acid and gamma linoleic acid. With regard to the butter versus margarine controversy it must be said that neither is a particularly recommended food. Butter contains excessive levels of saturated animal fats whereas margarine, although often made from plant oils, is so heavily manufactured that its nutritive properties are damaged. Margarine bears little resemblance to cold pressed plant oils, as these require hydrogenation to be converted into a solid. Vitamin E, which occurs naturally in all plant oils is often lost during the manufacturing process, creating a deficiency of this essential nutrient. Butter and margerine do, however, improve the flavour of many foods and may be considered indispensible in a bread eating society. They should therefore be used sparingly. For those who would like to give up both butter and margarine, nut butters made from peanuts, almonds or cashew nuts can be used on bread and are wholesome and nutritious.

Diet and the organs of elimination

At this point we must return to the core of the philosophy of natural medicine - the self-healing power of the human organism. A pre-requisite of biological life is that all organisms consume a nutritious food and expel the waste products via the organs of elimination. A natural diet of 70% fruit and vegetables and 30% small quantities of concentrated foods can be handled readily by the body. However, the western diet puts too great an emphasis on acid forming foods: meat, cheese, butter, milk, fried foods, soft drinks, tea, coffee, alcohol, etc. The waste products generated by this type of diet over burden the organs of elimination congesting the bloodstream and the arteries. These foods thereby become the main causative factor in heart disease, arterial damage, and other major diseases of modern society.

It is a contention in the philosophy of nature-cure that the accumulation of waste poisons in the system is the major starting point for many modern diseases. Anyone who would wish to remain healthy or build health would do well to assist the body's self-cleansing mechanism by drastically increasing their fruit and vegetable intake and cutting down heavily on concentrated foods. Short periods of an all fruit diet are immensely helpful. It might be mentioned here that catarrh is the body's own way of removing excessive waste poisons from the system. If the organs of elimination are over-run then the body ejects the waste products via mucous membranes. This is a safety mechanism and its action should not be discouraged. Cells die rapidly in a toxic acid bloodstream but thrive in a clean alkaline bloodstream. Anyone wishing to preserve youthfulness and vitality would therefore do well to recognise that the secret lies in a pure bloodstream which is fortified and nourished by the vitamins, minerals, proteins and trace elements that are provided by a natural diet.

White flour, salt and sugar

As stated earlier, man is the only animal to harness the use of fire for his own needs and as such is the only animal involved in the cooking of food. There is no question that heat destroys many of the living energies and nutrients in food and it is infinitely preferable to the digestive system and to one's health in general if food is eaten raw. Cooked food may be more appealing than raw, but this is purely an emotional sentiment borne largely out of habit and custom, rather than a physiological need. It is advisable therefore that as much raw food as possible be included in one's diet. As a general rule in the pursuit of health, certain foods ought to be omitted from the diet. These are white flour products, salt and sugar.

White flour begins its life as a wholegrain cereal which is then heavily processed to remove its fibre and wheatgerm. White flour is the result of a concentrated form of starch with the vitamins and minerals and fibre removed. Since many bowel and stomach disorders in western society are directly linked to a lack of dietary fibre, it would seem wise to substitute all white flour products with the real thing - wholewheat products. With regards to fibre in the diet, it ought to be mentioned that all plant foods contain fibre, animal foods none at all. This is a clear indication of the advisability of natural plant foods.

With regards to salt, there is little doubt that its excessive use is highly destructive. It is not only implicated in heart disease, hardening of the arteries and high blood pressure, but is particularly implicated as a major contributory factor in cancer. The main problem is that aside from the liberal use of salt sprinkled over most meats, salt is used extensively as a preservative and flavour enhancer in a great number of modern foods and drinks. In natural medicine, sodium (salt) free diets contribute a large part of the alternative treatment for cancer with much success. Sufficient salt occurs naturally in a plant food diet and it is not necessary, indeed inadvisable to include more in the diet.

White sugar is a highly refined carbohydrate and again widely over used in our society. It is implicated in many diseases of the western world, including obesity, diabetes, heart and circulatory disorders, hypoglycaemia and some mental disturbances, and its use ought to be severely restricted.

Towards a better diet

It is clearly advisable to avoid all junk foods and foods containing artificial additives, colourings or preservatives. Where possible, one should obtain organic foods grown without artificial sprays and pesticides. Natural foods can be inexpensive, since cereal grains, bean products and vegetables in season are relatively cheap. Protein from plant sources i.e. cereal grains, nuts, seeds and beans is quite sufficient to maintain health and if combined with low fat dairy products, would provide a nutritious wholesome diet.

A word can be mentioned here about three particular foods which are not only outstandingly nutritious but extremely inexpensive. Wheatgerm is the heart of the wheat kernel and is a store house of nutrients and essential fatty acids. It is a natural source of vitamins and minerals, particularly vitamin E and can be sprinkled on breakfast cereals or other foods. Brewers yeast is an immensely nutritious plant food containing 40% protein, many vitamins, minerals and enzymes, particularly 'B' complex, and is an outstanding natural tonic. Brewers yeast and wheatgerm when given to laboratory animals were shown to double their lifespan. The third food is blackstrap molasses which is loaded with vitamins, mineral salts and organic iron and can be taken off the spoon or made into a drink. These three foods are amongst the most nutritious available and possess great curative and health giving properties.

Other simple health-improving measures are as follows. Liquids and solids should not be consumed together at the same meal as the digestive juices required for the digestion of food are weakened by the intake of liquids. Liquids should be consumed either half an hour before or two hours after a meal. It has been suggested that mixing protein and starchy foods at the same meal is not conducive to sound digestive health and it may generally be wise to avoid combining too many different types of food at one meal.

The adoption of a plant food/raw food dietary regime (with some concessions to the intake of small quantities of animal foodstuffs, if considered necessary) would do much to eradicate many diseases of civilization. Raw food contains living energies not found in dead flesh, and passes on its life force to the health of the individual. The use of natural foods can slow down the ageing process to its minimum pace, import a healthy bloom to the complexion and can inspire the individual with positivity, vitality and a zest for life. Furthermore the use of natural foods and the observance of nature's laws would constitute the most significant stride towards the eradication of disease and ill-health from the midst of humanity.

As a final word on this subject it should be mentioned that 70% of the body's vitality and life-force is used up by the body's internal workings, (the circulation and digestion of food for example), and only 30% through physical activity. This is the reason that heavy meals are fatigue and sleep inducing. Food is converted by the vital force of the system into elements for energy and repair and as such, through the choice of small meals and eating what is required rather than what is desired, it is possible to liberate the body's life-force and vitality for the greater enjoyment of life's other interests. It is intended that the adoption of a natural food dietary regime should increase the vitality and well being of the individual, removing the spectre of illness and pain in order that life should become more enjoyable and pleasurable. Health and vitality are not the main aim in life, they are merely a pre-requisite to the enjoyment of life and are stepping stones in the pursuit of happiness and pleasure. After all, over whatever time scale, the gift of life would appear to have little other purpose than that it should be experienced and enjoyed to the full.

Masterwort
(Peucedanum Ostruthium)

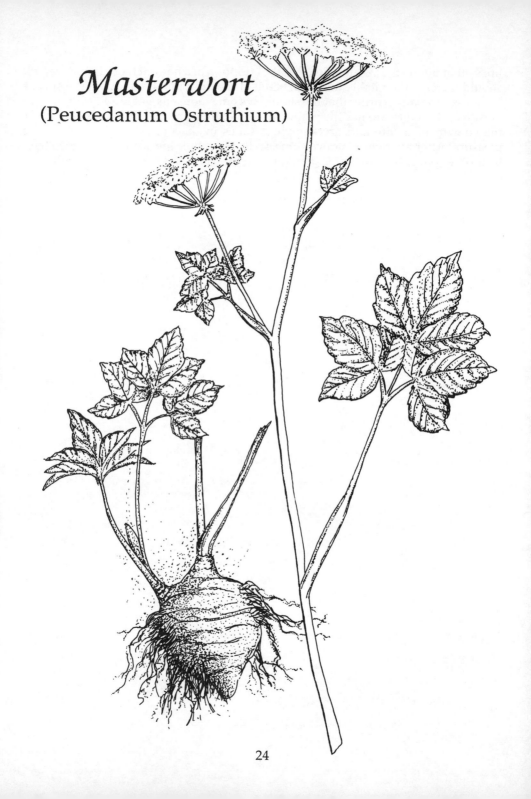

CHAPTER THREE

Cancer: Prevention and Cure

Each of us is composed of billions of cells which take in nutrients and expel waste products into the surrounding body fluids for elimination. These cells function in a highly controlled manner, working as a network with each group performing allotted tasks to maintain the physical equilibrium of the human organism. A cancerous growth occurs when a cell, or group of cells, cuts free from central control and commences to behave in an anti social fashion, reproducing rapidly at an uncontrolled rate, invading surrounding tissue, and often travelling the bloodstream, setting up colonies of malignant tumours. Cancer is feared more than any other western disease and for this reason a chapter is dedicated to to the illness here.

The orthodox medical approach to the growth of a cancerous tumour has changed little throughout the century in spite of billions of pounds spent annually researching a pharmaceutical solution. One wonders why this should be the case, but let us examine first the methods that are in use.

Surgery

Surgery, radiation and chemotherapy still constitute the main weapons of attack against cancer, an approach which comes in for some criticism from doctors and alternative practitioners alike. Surgical treatments of cancer involve amputation of the malignant growth, a procedure which is frequently valuable, not only because it allows time for the body's immune system to mobilise its defences but because it can frequently remove a life threatening condition. Criticism of this method of treatment is that it allows oxygen to get to the tumour and may contribute to a more rapid growth and spread throughout the system. Furthermore, surgery constitutes a stress factor to humans and can sap the body's vitality and strength, particularly the dynamism of the body's immune system which is involved in the control and destruction of cancerous cells. However, surgery can be successful in treating some forms of cancer and is the most commendable of the three treatments, though informed medical advice is necessary to evaluate its suitability in individual circumstances. What is certain, however, is that surgery does not pay any consideration whatsoever to the actual cause of the patient's cancer.

Radiotherapy

Radiotherapy pursues the same objective as surgery but it attempts to burn out the cancerous growth as opposed to surgical removal. Unfortunately, radiation destroys healthy cells as well as malignant ones, depletes the body's own natural resistance (the very system upon which the body depends in its fight against cancer) and is itself capable of rendering cells malignant rather than destroying them. Furthermore, the side effects of radiotherapy including chronic fatigue and exhaustion, nausea, weakness, loss of appetite and general sickness can be intolerable and dispiriting.

There is a widespread body of opinion which maintains that radiotherapy does little to improve the patient's chances of survival. The Swiss Institute for Experimental Cancer Research had this to say about the use of irradiation in breast cancer patients:

'In six controlled studies, survival rates were significantly lower amongst women who were irradiated than amongst those who were treated with surgery alone. Stopping the use of prophylactic local radiotherapy could increase survival rates'.

What is certain is that like surgery, radiation treatment does not respect the cause nor the circumstances of the individual's cancer.

Chemotherapy

Chemotherapy has even less to recommend it. This treatment involves the use of highly toxic drugs to destroy the malignant cells of the tumour. Unfortunately, these cyto-toxic drugs are non-selective and although they are successful in destroying cancerous cells they also destroy healthy cells. The cyto-toxic drugs are amongst the most toxic substances used in medicine and are also capable of inducing malignancy. Furthermore, the doses required for the destruction of cancerous cells are not much lower than the doses which are fatal to the healthy cells. The side effects of chemotherapy can be severe including anorexia, vomiting, nausea, renal disfunction, hair loss, liver and kidney damage, blood loss, diarrhoea, skin ulcers, mental confusion and severe emotional depression. Again, like radiotherapy, chemotherapy has a counter productive and debilitating action upon the body's natural defence system and pays no respect to the underlying causes of cancer.

Six million people still die of cancer world wide each year. In America alone one million people are under medical care at any one time for cancer. Of these 395,000 will die annually. The success or otherwise of orthodox treatments for cancer can best be summed up by Dr Ivon Illich:

'We do have increasing evidence that those who are treated for malignant disease, at best have an earlier onset of anguish, a prolonged period of impairment and a greater intensity of pain than those who succeed in escaping the doctor'.

Dr Hardin Jones of the University of California states: 'My studies have proven conclusively that untreated cancer victims actually live up to four or five times longer than treated individuals'.

The case of Jason Winters

If orthodox medical treatments are so unsuccessful in treating cancer, why should this be so and is there an alternative? As stated earlier billions of dollars have been spent researching a pharmaceutical solution for cancer, little if any of this money being spent on researching any nutritional considerations or investigating environmental causes. Alternative therapies which are always concerned with removing the cause of disease and liberating the body's self-healing capacity have likewise never been investigated. Also, as previously stated, it is estimated that one million Americans suffer from cancer at any one time, of these each is expected to spend approximately $25,000 in treatments. This makes cancer a billion dollar industry and may go some way to explaining the inertia of the medical authorities. The following true story may illuminate the situation further.

Jason Winters was 46 years and living in North America when he developed cancer. He underwent cobalt radiation treatment and used vitamin E oil to assist the healing of the burns on his face. The doctors remarked how well his radiation burns were improving with the vitamin E treatment but told him not to tell anyone about it. This puzzled Jason but the truth was to dawn as time passed on. The next day the surgeon informed Jason that he was to perform radical neck surgery, removing tongue, jaw bone and neck muscles, in an effort to arrest the spread of the disease. When the surgeon was asked whether this would lengthen his life, Jason was informed that it probably would not. On this note Jason left the surgery in pursuit of alternatives. He discovered the therapeutic action of laetrile (vitamin B17) which is extracted from apricot kernels and believed to have a specific anti-cancer action. Jason immediately bought six bottles of apricot kernels and consumed about fifty each day. His aches and pains stopped and the tumour appeared to be shrinking. When he returned to the health food store for more apricot kernels he was informed that the government authorities had removed them from the shelves. The explanation he received from the health food manager was that if vitamin B17 (Laetrile) was successful in treating cancer all those people involved in the cancer industry who make their living from the disease would suffer personal and financial hardship. Drug companies would lose millions of dollars annually, doctors, surgeons and anaesthetists would lose a lucrative part of their living and clinics and hospitals would be starved of their life blood. In brief Jason was forced to travel to Mexico for his laetrile treatments, where he experienced also the rejuvenating value of pure natural foods and positive thought. Within ten days his tumour had shrunk to half its normal size and he returned home with his laetrile tablets and presented himself for examination at his cancer clinic. Jason was anxious to see their response to his now almost completely disappeared tumour hoping for smiles and congratulations. Instead the doctor who had determined on radical surgery to the tongue and jaw bone proclaimed that Jason could never have had cancer in the first place. The doctors were neither particularly impressed nor particularly enthusiastic about Jason's apparent regression. Horrified by their attitude Jason left as quickly as possible.

In spite of a relapse soon afterwards, Jason was able to harness the forces of nature with other compounds, including laetrile, for a complete recovery from the disease.

The hounding of the professionals - Max Gerson

Throughout the last few decades practitioners and exponents of alternative treatments for cancer have been hounded and persecuted, particularly in America, by Government agencies and orthodox medicine. Many have been forced into bankruptcy through having to raise the money to defend themselves against repeated law suits and prosecution. Dr Max Gerson, one of the most respected pioneers of alternative cancer treatments had his membership to the American

Medical Society terminated, was unable to secure doctors to work with him and had to persistently fight to clear his methods of treatment in the law courts. What was his crime? He concentrated on removing the dietary causes of cancer, particularly excessive salt, and emphasised the importance of building up the constitution and the body's immune defence mechanism through the judicious use of nutritious foods. The reasons for the hostility of the AMS to Gerson's methods can best be summed up by an American cancer specialist of that era who said: "If this thing (the Gerson diet) works, we can chuck millions of dollars worth of equipment in the river and get rid of cancer by cooking carrots in a pot".

The causes of cancer

It was noted when kidney transplant patients were given drugs to suppress the action of the immune system from rejecting the kidney, many became increasingly susceptible to the onset of cancer. This is the clue that should give the reader a clear indication of the perspectives involved. The alternative or natural approach to cancer concentrates not on the cancer itself, but on the underlying causes that make cancer possible. Treatment is directed at bolstering the action of the body's resistance and invigorating the individual's immune system. Cancer rarely occurs in a healthy organism, it occurs largely when the individual's resistance and vitality are at a low ebb usually as a result of poor diet and unhealthy lifestyle. The approach is in keeping with the general philosophy of natural medicine which concerns itself with removing the cause of disease and allowing the body's restorative powers to flourish. The natural treatment for cancer is not unlike the natural treatment for most diseases, except that it is necessarily more intense and dynamic. When dealing with a cancer patient, the first step is to explore the possible reasons for the disease and to remove these from the individual's lifestyle, emphasising the importance of nature's healing forces in bolstering resistance.

What then is the immune defence mechanism? As part of the consequence of the gift of life, the human organism is vulnerable to the predatory action of the environment in the form of intrusive bacteria, carcinogens and viruses. The body's natural defence against these elements of danger is to form antibodies. Another feature of the immune system is the capacity of the body's white blood cells to move freely around the body taking action against unwelcome foreign agents, dissolving them into their own cytoplasm and removing the waste products. In this way, antibodies and white blood cells defend the individual's health, eliminating the cancer cell. It has been suggested that in the normal process of cellular reproduction, aberrant cells are frequently formed. In a healthy body these cells are overwhelmed and eliminated but where the immune system is below par or has been devitalised persistently by poor diet, stress, drugs and other unwholesome living habits, the immune system can be overrun and the pernicious onset of cancer triggered off.

Diet and cancer

In considering the causes of cancer and the predisposing influence of the immune system, it may be worthwhile to reflect once again on the lifestyle of the inhabitants of Hunza. They live in harmony with mother nature respecting her unwritten laws and dictates. They eat natural plant foods namely fruits, vegetables, nuts, seeds, beans and cereal grains, consume pure spring water, breathe fresh unpolluted mountain air, sleep 8-10 hours a night, work hard, pray and maintain a relaxed and unhurried approach to life. For this they are rewarded with a long life and a disease free existence. If we compare this with our own environment and our own lifestyles it is not too difficult to understand that the discrepancy between the two worlds illuminates the nature and causes of cancer. A brief consideration of this environmental aspect of cancer makes the medical treatments of radiation and chemotherapy seem all the more futile and misguided. The modern diet of the civilised west comprises a heavy consumption of animal foods with their excessive concentrations of animal fat and lack of fibre, canned and processed convenience foods, additives, preservatives, chemical sprays and pesticides, food dyes and colourings, fizzy drinks, alcohol, coffee and tobacco. Wholegrain cereals are stripped of their natural fibre and vitamins to create white flour - a food that is extensively used throughout society and extensively implicated in the onset of many diseases. Consider that in England and Wales 16,000 people die each year from cancer of the colon and rectum. In America the toll is 49,000 annually for the same disease, about one death every 10 minutes.

Digestion and cancer

Two British doctors, Burkitt and Trowell, discovered that the faecal matter passed by Africans was soft and bulky and that food passed through the body within 24 hours. By contrast the faecal matter of the British was hard, compressed and odiferous, taking three days to pass through the system. Since the Africans were largely free from cancer of the bowel and rectum it would seem to be particularly incumbent to assess the influence of their diet on their freedom from this form of cancer. The important factor was discovered to be vegetable fibre or roughage - the cellulose in plants which is indigestible but also indispensible in maintaining the health of the digestive system. Remember that animal foods contain no roughage or fibre. Wholegrain wheat begins its life as a nutritious fibre filled food but after heavy refining has removed its roughage, the wheatgerm is turned into fibreless white flour. It is perfectly clear that white flour products and the consumption of animal foods are seriously implicated in the development of cancer of the bowel and rectum.

Salt and cancer

Another major causative factor in cancer is the excessive use of sodium (salt) in the modern diet.

Dr Maud Tresilian Fere, a British doctor, cured herself of cancer using her own methods and explained these in her book *Cancer, its Dietetic Cause and Cure*. She maintains that body cells are influenced by their immediate environment and, in particular, that cancer cells are normal cells which have been forced to exist in the wrong body fluid environment. She maintains that the immune system is quite capable of keeping cancer cells in check unless there is an excess of sodium in the tissue fluids surrounding the cell. When this happens, the cancer cells multiply more rapidly in order to create lactic acid which can neutralise the action of excessive sodium. The cancer tumour is thus created by the effort of normal cells to protect themselves from excessive sodium. Whatever the complex mechanism behind the formation of the cancer cell, salt is certainly consumed excessively in the modern diet. It is used as a preservative in many processed and tinned foods, is included in many meats and their by products, is put in beer, bread, cheeses, modern medicines (aspirin for example) and is heavily used in butter, approximately half a teaspoon of salt occurs in 1oz of butter. Salt is, of course, also used extensively in cooking and is usually liberally applied from the salt pot. Whilst a small amount of salt in the diet is essential to health, sufficient is provided by a consumption of natural foods. It is estimated that the average individual consumes up to eight teaspoons of salt every 24 hours both from obvious and hidden sources. This level is certainly dangerous and ought to be strictly curtailed for cancer prevention and omitted totally in cancer treatment. Sodium free diets have been particularly favoured by alternative practitioners in the treatment of cancer and not surprisingly have enjoyed much success. In one study, animals fed on heavily salted cooked meat developed cancer within three months. When fed on raw unsalted meat the cancer regressed. Combined with an unhealthy diet, an excess of sodium contributes to the beginnings of cancer. Again it may become clear why orthodox treatment of cancer is incomplete. It may remove the growth but not the underlying condition which made the growth of the cancerous cell possible. Cancer is largely a constitutional disease and, if not treated with constitutional measures, is likely to recur elsewhere in the system.

Cigarettes and cancer

Another major cause of cancer is the self-inflicted use of tobacco. Lung cancer now causes 35% of cancer deaths in men. In 1978 the death toll from lung cancer amongst both sexes reached 100,000 in America the majority being cigarette smokers. Moreover, cigarette smokers run an increased risk of developing other forms of cancer, not to mention an increased risk of dying from heart disease. It has been estimated that each cigarette shortens the life span by 10 minutes.

Saturated fats and cancer

With regards to fats in the diet there is some evidence that an excessive use of both animal fats and polyunsaturated fats are equally undesirable in cancer prevention. Animal foods are natural only to carnivorous animals and so it is hardly surprising that animal fats should be injurious to health. Polyunsaturated fats from plant foods are essential to health but should be obtained from their food sources of nuts, seeds, beans, wheatgerm, olives, avocados, etc. When it was first determined that polyunsaturated fats could reduce blood cholesterol levels, some devotees were drinking these oils by the bottle. Nature requires more subtlety than this, one tablespoon daily being all that is required. The oils in plant foods contain vitamin E, a vitally important nutrient much of which is lost if the plant oils are extracted with heat. Lack of vitamin E can cause premature ageing, wrinkles and loose skin and can predispose towards heart and circulatory disorders. For this reason it may be wise, if margarine and polyunsaturated oils are used extensively, to take a vitamin E capsule daily.

It is particularly important that polyunsaturated oils should not be allowed to go rancid because they can produce a potent carcinogen (cancer forming agent) called malonaldehyde. Oils should therefore be bought in small quantities, preferably cold pressed and kept refrigerated. The temptation to heat oils to high temperatures for the purpose of frying foods is also an unwelcome habit. Polyunsaturates ought to be provided naturally in the diet from food sources, or used in the form of cold pressed oil wich can be used in salad dressings, olive oil probably being best. The equivalent of one tablespoon from food, or as a supplement, is all that is needed daily.

Low protein intakes tend to correlate with low incidences of cancer as any study of primitive races of healthy inhabitants will show. The Hunzas consume about 50 grams of vegetable protein daily. Mormons and Seventh Day Adventists both observe healthy lifestyles and have low incidences of disease. The Adventists, however, are vegetarians and experience a much lower cancer rate than the meat-eating Mormons.

Sugar and cancer

Dr John Judkin, a foremost authority on the harmful action of sugar on the body maintains that excessive consumption of this food may well increase the likelihood of the development of malignant tumours It is a concentrated form of starch which is excessively over used, lacks roughage and provides calories without any nutrients. Not only this but sugar depletes essential nutrients in the system including magnesium, zinc, chromium and many of the 'B' vitamins. Most importantly, however, sugar has been shown to have a detrimental and devitalising action upon the effectiveness of the immune system. It appears to interfere with the capacity of the white blood cells to overcome intrusive organisms, rendering the individual more susceptible to the onset of cancer. Also, as sugar is implicated in diseases of the circulatory system, it would seem wise to reduce this element to an absolute minimum, paying particular attention to the hidden foods in which it occurs.

Water and cancer

Modern society makes use of many thousands of chemicals of which the National Cancer Institute maintains that approximately 1,000 are potentially carcinogenic. Water pollutants are believed to contain some danger to the individual, for example lead, arsenic, nickel and particularly cadmium appear to have a link with cancer. Fluoride added to water in large amounts has increased the growth of tumours in laboratory animals and this itself is a possible cause of concern. It should also be mentioned that cancer patients on a sodium-free diet should avoid water to which sodium fluoride has been added, as this is clearly another form of salt. It may be wise to consume bottled spring water when possible.

Drugs, X-rays and cancer

Many common drugs can contribute towards cancer. Dr Roger Williams cites Reserpine (a drug used to cure high blood pressure) as being conceivably responsible for 5,000 cancer cases each year. Excessive use of X-rays has also been implicated. A commission on radiology in America indicated that X-ray treatments in the USA produce 3,000 deaths a year from various forms of cancer and genetic damage. What is more no-one knows for sure what the legacy of the present use of X-rays will be for future generations. Clearly it is important to avoid as many carcinogenic substances as possible, though due to the complexity of the modern technological age with the consequent pollution of air, food and water, this is not easy.

The solution

Considering the number of carcinogens to which we are all continuously subjected, it is surprising that the human race manages to survive at all. But survive it does. In spite of the number of people who die from cancer, most do not. Of those exposed to a virulent carcinogen, only a small percentage will succumb to cancer, the rest will remain resistant. Herein lies the solution to the dilemma. The critical factor is not so much the antagonist as the quality of the individual's resistance, not so much the cancer cell as the immune system's power to overcome it. A natural treatment will therefore provide natutral immunity.

The first step in the treatment of cancer is to remove all junk foods, additives and preservatives, all animal foods, salt, sugar, tea, coffee and alcohol from the diet and replace these with pure, natural foods, comprising solely of plant foods, fruits, vegetables, nuts, seeds, beans and cereal grains, preferably organically grown and eaten raw. Heavy emphasis is placed on fruits, vegetables and their juices due to their invigorating action upon the immune system and also to their high content of potassium which removes excessive sodium from the diet. The aim of the early stages of cancer treatment is to both fortify the immune system through the choice of a raw plant food diet and to assist the body in its efforts to detoxify the poisons which have accumulated in the body due to previous excesses.

The action of the body in continuously cleansing itself of the toxins generated by food and oxygen intake has been mentioned previously. It is a major function of all life forms that after nutrients have been extracted from food the waste products generated should be removed from the body via the eliminatory organs: the lungs, the skin and the bowels. Because of the concentrated nature of the modern diet which emphasises a heavy indulgence in animal proteins, starch and fatty foods, the organs of elimination frequently struggle to cope with the build up of waste poisons in the system. A diet of natural plant foods releases the body's self-cleansing mechanism, thus removing toxins and their deleterious action on the individual's health, from the system.

It must be remembered that the cancer diet is not a special diet, it is purely a natural diet which all would benefit greatly from adhering to. It is not a temporary diet, it is a healthful diet of natural foods which mother nature intended us to consume for our greater benefit and well-being.

A further theory in the treatment of cancer, and part of the reasons for the omission of meat from the diet, is that the pancreas produces pancreatic enzymes which are involved with the digestion of protein. If meat is consumed then the pancreatic enzymes are side-tracked towards the digestion of meat rather than towards the destruction of the tumorous growth. One peculiar feature of the cancer cell is that it is coated with protein which enables it to evade the body's immune system. It is considered that this protein coating can be stripped by pancreatic enzymes leaving the cancerous cell more vulnerable to eradication. For this reason a low protein diet is observed, sufficient only to stimulate the pancreas to produce its protein digesting enzymes. As cooking destroys vital nutrients all food should be consumed raw as nature intended.

The next aspect of the cancer treatment is the decisive use of certain vitamins and minerals for their action in stimulating the immune system. The following list covers the most commonly accepted of these.

Natural Treatments

Vitamin B17 (Laterile)

Laetrile, or vitamin B17, has aroused raging controversy in the West with proponents of natural therapies in cancer proclaiming its miraculous virtues and opponents (usually the orthodox medical societies) denouncing it vehemently and attempting with much success to ban its use. What is more, primitive societies that consume foods high in nitrilosides (vitamin B17) appear to have a strong degree of protection against cancer. The Hunzas for one consume large quantities of apricot kernels which are the most profuse source of nitrilosides. Eskimos living largely on meat are also free of cancer, due, it appears, to the fact that the animals they kill have fed on nitriloside rich food. In this way they obtain their B17 second hand. The meat diet of the Eskimos does lead to degenerative diseases but cancer is largely absent. The rural inhabitants of the Philippines and West Indies, although consuming large quantities of a poor quality food called Cassava nevertheless have low incidences of cancer, due to its high vitamin B17 content. Where

the diet is vegetarian, well balanced and high in nitriloside rich foods there is generally good health, longevity and freedom from cancer. Where the diet is poor, yet rich in vitamin B17 the lifespan is shorter but cancer does still not appear. In primitive days man would have consumed large quantities of nitriloside rich food which would have offered protection against cancer, but in the present day, due to the consumption of modern foods and modern processing methods, there is an almost total lack of these vital nitrilosides in the typical diet. If vitamin B17 is considered to be a true vitamin then cancer may be seen as a deficiency disease on an epidemic scale, treatable in much the same way as other deficiency diseases.

Laetrile is the proper name for the purified crystallised concentrate of vitamin B17 and is used not as a preventative but as a major anti cancer agent. It can be broken down into three basic elements: sugar, benzaldehyde and hydrogen cyanide. These elements can selectively destroy cancer cells and can be included in the diet in the form of apricot kernels. However, there is only a small amount of B17 in these kernels and the amount that would need to be consumed orally is prohibitive due to their cyanide content which can induce sickness. Laetrile, the concentrate of vitamin B17, is preferred because this can be taken in tablet or injection form allowing larger quantities of vitamin B17 to be taken. The great value of laetrile lies largely in its ability to be selective and non-injurious to normal cells. It should be remembered that chemotherapy drugs are destructive of both cancerous and normal body cells, whereas laetrile can be used extensively and for an indefinite period without side effects. When laetrile reaches the cancerous cell it is broken down into its three nitriloside compounds, sugar, benzaldehyde and hydrogen cyanide, the last two being extremely poisonous to cancer cells. Other research has shown that thiocyanate, a substance derived from one of the nitrilosides, can remove the protective protein coat of the cancer cell thus rendering the cell defenceless to invasion by white body cells. It must be stressed here that the use of laetrile is likely to be more successful when combined with a full anti-cancer regime. It is not a miracle cure, but when combined with the action of alternative treatments in boosting the body's immune system, results have been very positive. As a preventative of cancer it would seem prudent to include nitriloside rich foods in the diet.

Foods high in nitrilosides

Seeds and beans are particularly high in nitrilosides, especially when sprouted and they should form the main part of an anti-cancer diet.

To sprout seeds, soak them first for several hours. Spread the seeds on a sprouting tray, a dish or in a glass jar and place in a darkened atmosphere at room temperature. Rinse the seeds twice daily. When the sprouts appear (usually between 3-4 days) bring into the light and continue the twice daily rinsing routine. Eat when the sprouts are approximately one inch long.

The following foods are particularly high in B17, especially when sprouted.

Seeds and beans
Alfalfa
Millet
Mung beans
Lentils
Bitter almonds

Fruit and vegetable seeds
Apple seeds
Apricot kernels (These resemble almonds in appearance and taste).
Cherry pits
Nectarine pits
Peach pits
Prune pits
Pear seeds

(The stones can be cracked with a nut-cracker and the pits eaten whole or ground.)

Others
The following are moderately high in nitrilosides:
Buckwheat
Linseed
Millet
Raspberries
Blackberries
Elderberries
The following contain some B17 though not high doses
Broccoli
Cabbage
Cauliflower
Spinach
Sweet Potato

Watercress
Barley
Oats
Rye
Black Eyed Beans
Chick Peas
Green Peas
Cashew Nuts
Brown Rice

The B17 of those items in the first group is above 500mg per 100 gms. The third group contains 100mg per 100 grams and the second group lies between these two ranges.

It must be mentioned that laetrile can only be obtained from a medical practitioner sympathetic to alternative treatments. Laetrile can be obtained from Cantassium Larkhall Labs, 229 Putney Bridge Road, London, but only with a note from the practitioner taking responsibility for the injections. A word should be mentioned here about the *Bristol Cancer Help Centre* set up in the early 1980s and now greatly expanded due to the pressure of increased demand. Anyone wishing to turn to alternative methods of cancer treatment ought to contact this organisation and ask them to send the introductory package on the Bristol Cancer Centre treatment, which will include a tape, several booklets and general information about the Clinic. Visitors to the Clinic are encouraged, where they will receive a warm welcome and much moral support. Longer term patients are accepted. The address is: Bristol Cancer Centre, Grove House, Cornwallis Grove, Bristol, Tel. 0272 736226. Treatment is under the professional guidance of Dr Alec Forbes, a founder member of the Clinic.

Treatment for any cancer should be undertaken only under the guidance of a qualified medical practitioner. No claims can be made for laetrile except that when combined with a holistic approach to cancer with particular emphasis upon a natural dietary regime, it appears to assist the body to gain control of an existing cancer. Vitamin B17 may also be included in the diet in the form of nitriloside rich foods, as part of an overall programme of dietary and lifestyle improvements in the prevention of cancer.

Vitamin C

Professor Linus Pauling a nobel prize winner for his efforts in the field of science and an eminent authority on vitamin C maintains that the use of this nutrient increases the body's production of collagen which has the capacity of strengthening the intercellular cement which holds normal body cells together, rendering them more resistant to damage from cancer cells. In controlled studies in a Glasgow hospital it was shown that vitamin C in doses of 10 grams daily improved the state of well being of the patients, relieved their pain and increased their life spans considerably. Some patients experienced complete remissions and were still alive several years after the experiments. Linus Pauling maintains that there is much evidence that increasing the intake of vitamin C significantly decreases the chances of the individual developing cancer. Vitamin C has anti-stress properties and stimulates the body's production of lymphocytes which are involved as part of the body's defence mechanism. At the Bristol Cancer Centre high doses of vitamin C are used, about 6 grams daily, combined with bioflavonoids which always occur with vitamin C in nature. This treatment has the action of invigorating the body's immune system and detoxifying toxic substances which enter the bloodstream, including carcinogens. Due to the shortage of vitamin C in modern foods and to the fact that primitive man would have obtained several thousand milligrams of vitamin C daily from his food it may be wise to take Professor Pauling's advice and include several grams of vitamin C as a supplement in the daily diet.

Vitamin A

This is also believed to exert an invigorating action on the immune system and is included extensively in the Bristol Cancer programme provided largely by intakes of fresh carrot juice up to 1.5 pints daily. Vitamin A is believed to assist the action of B17 in its destruction of tumours and has a protective and therapeutic action in general against particular forms of cancer.

Vitamin E

This nutrient maintains healthy blood vessels, is an anti blood-clotting agent and is useful in the treatment and prevention of heart and circulatory disorders. Vitamin E is also an anti-oxidant which reduces the severity of oxygen and free radicals in ageing the cells of the body. This process needs a brief explanation.

Metals tend to rust in the presence of oxygen

and similarly an apple halved will soon begin to deteriorate when exposed to the air. The modern environment is particularly high in corrosive oxidants found largely in the air, in atmospheric pollution and frequently in food and water. It is believed that these cause the body to rust and age at a faster rate than normal. Certain nutrients appear to display a specific antioxidant action, vitamin C and selenium in particular, but the most potent anti oxidant of all is vitamin E. Animals given vitamin E could withstand the effects of environmental pollutants up to 100% longer than animals with inadequate intakes of vitamin E. An experiment was then conducted to see if anti oxidants and vitamin E in particular could protect cells from damage caused by carcinogens (cancer-forming agents). Vitamin C reduced the cellular damage by 31.7%, selenium by 41% and vitamin E by 63.2%. The ability of vitamin E to protect the cell from the ravages of oxidants and carcinogens is the principal reason for its use in an anti-cancer programme. Between 500i.u's and 800 i.u's are taken daily but this should be under medical supervision. Vitamin E is not recommended for people with cancer of the female reproductive organs.

Selenium

This is an important nutrient in the cancer programme, due also to its anti-oxidant properties and the protection it affords the cell from oxidants and carcinogens. Selenium is irregularly distributed throughout the earth's soils, and epidemiological evidence shows that people living in high selenium areas have lower levels of cancer than those living in low selenium areas. In the UK, Norfolk shows high selenium levels in the soil and has a low incidence of cancer. Studies of 34 American cities again confirm that high selenium levels in the diet corresponded with low cancer rates, the lowest rate occurring in Rapid City, South Dakota, which had the highest selenium rate of all the cities involved. Laboratory experiments on animals showed that increasing their selenium levels had a marked impact on the animals natural resistance to cancer, their production of antibodies being significantly increased. A report in *Prevention* magazine commented that in a study of 1,000 people, those with the lowest levels of selenium in their blood had the highest incidences of cancer. Selenium is clearly a vital nutrient in any anti-cancer regime, though it is not necessary, indeed not advisable that it should be taken in high doses. Supplements of selenium are best absorbed in the form of organic selenium yeast 100 mcgs to 200 mcgs daily being all that is required. Natural sources of selenium should also be included in the diet, principally brewers yeast and wheatgerm.

Zinc

This mineral is frequently lacking in the modern diet due to the prevalence of poor quality crops grown on zinc deficient soils and to the destructive activity of food processing and refining. Wholewheat flour, for example, loses 78% of its zinc in the process of conversion into white flour. Alcohol and sugar consumption may further deplete the body's stores of this mineral. Zinc is believed to be necessary in the diet for the production of lymphocytes in particular and for the optimum healthy functioning of the body's immune system in general. The Bristol Cancer Help Centre recommends zinc orotate 100mg tablets to be taken, one daily is all that is required.

Magnesium

As with selenium, when soil magnesium levels are high, incidences of cancer and heart disease are low. When magnesium levels fall, incidences of cancer and heart disease increase. In Egypt where the cancer rate was shown in the past to be only one tenth that of the Europeans, it was discovered that they were consuming five or six times more magnesium than their European counterparts. Similar results have been found in experiments on animals. As with zinc, magnesium is easily lost in the process of refining. White bread for example has lost 85% of its natural magnesium.

Dolomite

The Bristol Cancer Help Centre recommends Dolomite as a supplement which contains both magnesium and calcium in the correct balance. Use is also made of magnesium and calcium supplements in orotic acid form. Orotic acid is vitamin B13 and is combined with mineral supplements in order to increase its absorption into the bloodstream. Natural sources of magnesium are wheatgerm, wholegrain cereals, bananas, molasses, beans and nuts and seeds.

Potassium

This is an important nutrient for the cancer patient as it has the ability to take excess sodium out of the body. This nutrient is best supplied by raw fruits and vegetables and their juices.

Iodine

A deficiency of this nutrient is believed to be a contributory factor in the development of breast cancer. It is needed in only tiny amounts and is specifically involved in the health of the thyroid gland. A deficiency is unlikely on a natural diet but it may be wise to take some kelp (seaweed) tablets which are a natural source of this element. Other minerals which are necessary for their protective action against cancer are molybdenum and chromium which again are heavily destroyed in the processing and refining of foods. Molybdenum occurs in natural foods like beans, wholegrain cereals and leafy vegetables. Chromium is found in fruits and vegetables and particularly in brewers yeast.

If the use of individual mineral supplements seem impractical and prohibitive due to the large numbers of supplements that would require to be taken, it may be best to take a high quality multi-mineral, preferably in orotate form, which contains some of all of these essential minerals. To this could be added organic selenium yeast (100 mcg once daily) and zinc orotate (100mg once daily). Kelp and dolomite could also be included. Professional advice and supervision is required and this could be obtained from the Bristol Cancer Help Centre, a qualified practitioner or other alternative cancer clinics.

Other nutritional supplements in the cancer programme include the following.

Bromelain - this is a digestive enzyme extracted from pineapple. It is credited (like the pancreatic enzymes released by the pancreas) with the ability to de-shield the protective protein coating of the cancer cell rendering it open to attack by the immune system. Dose: one 100mg tablet taken 4 times daily before meals, this dose being gradually increased.

Ginseng is frequently administered as it boosts the immune system and is a natural source of plant steroids.

Evening Primrose Oil capsules are taken also for their high content of Gamma Linoleic Acid (GLA) which has the action of stimulating prostaglandins noted for their ability to inhibit the growth of cancer cells.

Herbs are frequently used for their action in stimulating the liver in its work of detoxifying the poisons generated by the destruction of cancerous matter. Dandelion root, gentian root, burdock root, echinacea root and holy thistle leaves are some of the plants used. Due to the complexity of these treatments, particularly for those uninitiated in the art of alternative therapies it is incumbent that they seek professional advice and counselling before commencing these treatments. Once the treatments have been practiced and understood it will be possible to continue them from home. Of course it should go without saying that observance of all of nature's eight healing forces is paramount in building up the individual's constitution. Sleep, rest, exercise, sunshine and fresh air are all vitally important health building measures in any anti-cancer regime. There is however one healing force which requires special attention.

Positive thought / emotional poise

There is little doubt that an important factor in the development of cancer and its treatment is to be found in the emotional and spiritual condition of the patient. Negative emotions can suppress the action of the body's immune system whereas positive thoughts and feelings have the opposite action and invigorate the activity of the body's natural defences. It was noted many years ago in Ancient Greece that melancholia was more likely to be a component of the cancer patient's personality than optimism. As long ago as 1846 the following passage appeared in a book, *The Nature and Treatment of Cancer* and is worth repeating here.

'Much has been written on the influence of mental misery, sudden reverses of fortunes and habitual gloominess of temper on the deposition of carcinomatous matter, which would seem to constitute the most powerful cause of this disease. Morbid emotions produce defective innervation and this causes a perversion of nutrition which in turn causes the formation of carcinoma. Although the influence of mental disquietude has never been made a matter for demonstration it would be vain to deny facts of a very convincing character in respect to the agency of the mind in the production of this disease. I have met with cases in which the connection appeared so clear that to question its reality would have seemed to struggle against reason.'

It has been widely recognised that the onset of cancer is quite often preceded by some great shock or emotional trauma and upheaval in the individual's life, sometimes occurring two or three years prior to the development of the disease. Where possible the cancer sufferer should abandon passive submission to their disease in favour of confidence, determination, aggression and a firm resolve that with a prolonged and sustained attack from the combined powers of mind and body, they can drive their disease vigorously out of their system. Positive thought and an optimistic disposition can increase the levels of gamma globulin in the blood which is an important indication of the dynamism of the immune system. It is clear that a positive stance in the face of adversity can exert a profound influence upon the individual's neuro-endocrine system to their own advantage. Dr Carl Simonton took the influence of the mind in cancer treatment one step further. He discovered through his investigations of cancer patients who had recovered from their disease that they tended to share similar qualities of character, positivity and determination. He wondered whether patients who were less highly motivated against their disease could be encouraged to master certain mental techniques which would stimulate the immune system into action. Thus was borne the Simonton Visualisation Technique. In this method patients are taught to look into their own bodies and visualise the destruction of the cancerous tumour by the immune defence mechanism. The patient can use whatever images of antagonism they prefer, but the end result of overwhelming the cancerous tumour will remain consistent. For the individual with serious emotional difficulties which interfere with the body's self-healing progress psychotherapeutic help will be needed at the hands of an experienced practitioner.

The Bristol Cancer Help Centre places great emphasis upon the psychological, emotional and spiritual condition of the cancer sufferer and it would clearly be wise to visit the clinic in order to gain a fuller understanding of these therapies.

The alternative treatment of cancer as elucidated in these pages can clearly be seen as a 'holistic' approach operating on all levels, mind, body and spirit in an effort to stem the tide of cancer in our midst and to encourage the individual back to glorious health.

It would certainly be wise to avoid as many environmental carcinogens as possible in the prevention and treatment of cancer. Here follows a list of the most prominent according to Dr Isaac Bryant in his book *'Cancer, the Alternative Method of Treatment'*.

1 Smoking

2 Occupational pollutants

3 Sunlight and X-radiation

4 Pesticides, growth hormones, food additives

5 Water pollution, especially chlorine and fluorides

6 Undernutrition and lack of fibre

7 Air pollution

8 Heavy drinking of alcohol

9 Some drugs used in medicines

10 Negative or suppressed emotions

Avoidance of these carcinogenic factors should be complemented by the adoption of all health building measures which invigorate the immune system and fortify the individual against the ravages of the environment. Only in this way, through respect for the laws of the universe and humility before nature can the spectre of cancer be removed from our midst.

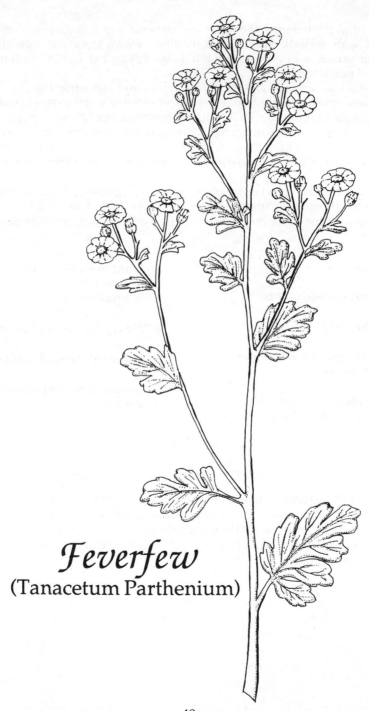

Feverfew
(Tanacetum Parthenium)

CHAPTER FOUR

Heart and Circulation

D iseases of the heart and circulation have reached epidemic proportions in America, Great Britain and other western civilised countries over the last few decades. It was estimated in the 1960s that over ten million Americans suffered from diseases of the heart and circulation and that almost one million of these could expect to die annually. In Great Britain in 1982 40% of all male deaths were caused by diseases of the heart and arteries and 38% of all female deaths. Heart disease in Great Britain claims 200,000 lives each year, approximately one death every three minutes. There are now more deaths from heart and circulatory disorders in Britain per head of population than anywhere in the world, with Scotland, Wales and Northern Ireland being the countries worst affected. Furthermore, diseases of the heart and circulation are not confined purely to the elderly. In a study of 300 American soldiers killed in the Korean war, it was found that 77% showed deposits of cholesterol and plaque in their arteries, due principally to their heavy consumption of cholesterol rich animal foods. However in the Korean soldiers whose diet was largely vegetarian, no signs of arterial disease were evident. In order to understand better the causes of heart and circulatory disease it is important to explore briefly the role of the blood and circulation in maintaining the health of the body.

The bloodstream carries oxygen and nutrients to the cells and removes their waste products. It regulates the heart beat, carries hormonal secretions around the body and is the transport system of the immune defence mechanism. The circulation itself is motivated by the regular pumping action of the heart which contracts and relaxes at rhythmic intervals forcing blood through the large sophisticated network of arteries, veins and capillaries. The heart beats on average 70 times per minute, about 37 million times a year. It is the most highly sophisticated pump ever devised and is responsible for forcing 2,000 gallons of blood around the human system every 24 hours. If the role of the heart is to pump blood around the circulatory system then it depends upon the arteries of the body to fulfill this role. The arteries (tubes of smooth, soft elastic muscle tissue) carry the blood with its oxygen and nutrients to feed every cell and every part of the body. These arteries then subdivide into smaller arteries and finally into minute hairlike blood vessels known as capillaries. Capillaries stretch over thousands of miles in the human body and in spite of their microscopic size, each capillary being only one fiftieth of the width of a human hair, they allow the passage of blood corpuscles in single file along their microscopic corridors to feed the body cells with nutrients and oxygen and to carry away their waste products. In normal circumstances this complicated and highly sophisticated network of arteries, veins and capillaries orchestrated by the action of the heart, works in a well organised and effective manner. However, due to the dietary excesses and poor habits of living prevalent in modern man, this perfectly synchronised system is placed under considerable stress. When the arteries of the healthy individual are soft and pliable they can contract and expand easily when forcing blood along their corridors, but when these arteries become hard and brittle with deposits of fat and cholesterol accumulating on the arterial wall, this narrowing of the arterial corridor invariably inhibits the flow of blood. This can then lead to a raising of the blood pressure with the heart being required to work harder to force the blood around the system. If the artery becomes narrowed further by cholesterol deposits developing along its interior walls then eventually a blood clot may form, obstructing the circulation of the blood completely. If this occurs in an artery feeding the brain then what is commonly known as a 'stroke' will occur. When this happens, the part of the brain which is deprived of its blood supply will cause paralysis of that part of the body which it controls. Recovery depends upon whether the clot can be re-absorbed. If this is not the case, the part of the brain which has been deprived of oxygen and nutrients will be permanently damaged with the paralysis of the body similarly permanent. If an artery which supplies blood to the heart becomes congested and narrowed with fatty cholesterol deposits then ultimately a blood clot may form obstructing the circulation and depriving the heart muscle of its oxygen and nutrients. When this happens, what is commonly known as a 'heart attack' takes place.

Coronary heart disease is caused by narrowing or hardening of the coronary arteries - those arteries which supply the heart with blood and consequently the body's essential supply of nutrients and oxygen. When these coronary arteries become congested and the supply of blood to the heart is impaired, the disease progresses and chest pain, sometimes excruciating, will result. This is known as Angina, or 'Angina Pectoris', and occurs when one of the coronary arteries goes into spasm as a result of an inadequate oxygen supply. These attacks normally last only several minutes but if extended over a long period a coronary thrombosis (heart attack) must be suspected. Although heart disease and heart attacks in particular may appear to strike with great suddenness there is little doubt that the predisposing factor, narrowing and obstruction of the walls of the arteries, occurs over a protracted period of time.

However, heart disease and arterial damage are not exempt from the capacity of the body to heal itself. If an artery becomes obstructed with plaques of fat and cholesterol, that part of the heart which is deprived of oxygen and nutrients dies. However the body immediately begins to repair the damage, dead tissue being carried away from the affected part and built up with scar tissue. New blood vessels are frequently formed to carry out the work of the obstructed artery. If the sufferer from heart disease recognises the self rejuvenating power of the body, and accepts the need for a prolonged period of rest and rehabilitation with emphasis upon removing the causes of his/her disease and rebuilds the constitution with judicious respect to the forces of nature, then recovery can be markedly anticipated.

In exploring the causes of heart and circulatory troubles, it has been said that diseases of the arteries come to all who live long enough. This is not true. As people grow older, blood vessels do appear to lose their elasticity though this is not due to the effects of ageing but rather due to habits of living. It is possible to maintain the health and elasticity of the blood vessels and arteries and to prevent the arteries furring with fat and cholesterol if the body is treated properly and fed on the proper foods observing the fundamental rules of nature.

As stated earlier, due to man's long evolutionary development on a diet of fruits, nuts and seeds and vegetables, it should not be surprising that animal fats from flesh foods and dairy products are so injurious to health. Animal fats are saturated fats and have little nutritional value and are damaging to the system. Plant oils, however, from nuts, seeds, beans, wheat-germ, olives, avocados etc. provide unsaturated fatty acids which are vitally important nutrients and which are essential to health. These unsaturated fatty acids, or polyunsaturated fatty acids, are beneficial in treating and preventing skin complaints, including eczema, are useful in premenstrual tension due to their action of stimulating hormones (prostaglandins), in preventing thrombosis and most pointedly in reducing high blood cholesterol levels. It is now accepted that high blood cholesterol levels created by a diet high in saturated animal fats are a predisposing factor in heart disease. In world wide surveys it is always established without exception that populations with a low intake of animal fat have low incidences of atherosclerosis (fat deposits in the arteries). Japanese people when adhering to their normal diet of rice, vegetables and sea-food have extremely low incidences of heart and arterial disease, but on adopting western diets their coronary and artery disease rates become the same as those in the western world.

It should be noted that the philosophy of natural medicine throughout history has always maintained that heart and circulatory diseases are caused principally by faulty nutrition and in particular by the congestion of the bloodstream with toxic wastes generated by the consumption of concentrated animal foods. Nature-cure practitioners (Naturopaths) have adopted this stance throughout the century by observing man in his environment and by recognising the laws of nature. The first step in the prevention or treatment of heart disease and arterial degeneration should be to maintain the bloodstream in a clean, well-nourished, toxin free condition. This can be achieved through the adoption of a plant food diet comprising fruits, vegetables, nuts, seeds, beans and cereal grains. Low fat dairy products and small quantities of lean animal foods, fish or chicken for example, could be included if thought necessary.

It would seem to be beyond credibility that medical research is directed towards the discovery of drugs and medicines to placate the symptoms of heart and circulatory diseases rather than to promote the cleansing of the arteries and bloodstream through the choice of pure food and water. In his book *Food for a Future*, Jon Wynne Tyson creates the analogy that using medicines to treat diseases of the heart and arteries is akin to poisoning a river with sewage and industrial poisons and attempting to cure this with medication. The cure is quite evidently to stop polluting the river with poisons and allow it to regain its former crystal clear health.

However, reducing animal fats in the diet and adopting wholesome eating habits in the prevention and treatment of circulation disorders does require further elucidation. Hardening of the arteries may well develop partly as a result of consuming cholesterol rich foods but also partly as a result of a constitutional debility and disharmony which may cause faulty utilisation of these fats. Certain hormones which normally break up fatty foods are often lacking in those people suffering from circulatory diseases, notably thyroid hormones. Furthermore animal fats are not the only food factors implicated in heart disease. A heavy consumption of sugars and starches in the diet can lead to an accumulation of fats in the blood and predispose the body to arterial damage.

In general, it is important to see heart disease and hardening of the arteries as a constitutional disorder brought about by general debilitating factors in the individual's lifestyle rather than just by an excessive consumption of animal fats. The effects of tobacco for example should not be dismissed. Men under 45 who smoke 25 cigarettes a day on average have fifteen times the risk of developing heart disease than non-smokers. Cigarette smoking makes a significant contribution to hardening of the arteries. The consumption of a diet high in junk foods, sugars, salt, chemical fertilisers, preservatives, colouring, additives, processed foods, coffee and alcohol are likely to have an accumulative effect in contributing towards heart disease and degeneration of the arteries. Foods which congest the bloodstream, principally the concentrated foods classified as fats, proteins or carbohydrates, as opposed to the cleansing, foods of fruit and vegetables are likely to predispose one to heart disease or arterial damage if consumed to excess. A strong effort should be made then to keep the bloodstream clean through a heavy emphasis upon fruits and vegetables (70%) and small quantities (30%) of foods from other groups (fat, carbohydrate, proteins), though these should be from plant food rather than animal sources.

The absence of roughage in the diet also plays a significant role in the development of arterial disease. This can be corrected by excluding animal foods which contain no fibre from the diet and emphasising plant foods which contain fibre without exception. White flour products should be avoided as these have had the fibre removed.

Stress undoubtedly plays a significant role due to its debilitating action on the system in general and the nervous system in particular. An effort should be made to secure plenty of sleep and rest, to approach life in a more relaxed and phlegmatic fashion and to develop techniques of deep relaxation either through yoga or meditation. Exercise should not be forgotten as this oxygenates the blood, invigorates the whole circulation and improves the body's metabolism.

Finally, as it is clear that heart and arterial disease are brought about principally by an excessive consumption of fatty foods and rich foods and by the inability of an impaired constitution to break down these fatty deposits a breakdown will be included in this chapter on specific foods, vitamins, minerals and fatty acids which have a tonic action in general and a specific action in particular in preventing and alleviating diseases of the heart and circulation.

Polyunsaturated fatty acids

These have been mentioned earlier in their capacity to reduce high cholesterol levels. These essential fatty acids can be obtained from their food sources of nuts, seeds (sunflower seeds) and beans (soya beans etc.) or as oil of evening primrose which has a specifically high concentration of Gamma Linoleic Acid. Olive oil can be used as a salad dressing preferably in cold pressed form. It is not recommended to use vegetable oils that have been heated to high temperatures as this destroys many of their properties.

Fish Oils

These have a particular protective action against heart and circulatory disease. These fish oils occur in fatty fish like herring, mackerel and salmon and are known as the Omega 3 fatty acids comprising two special essential fatty acids eicosapentaenoic acid (EPA) and docosahexaenoic acid (DPA). These fatty acids do not occur in vegetable oils and function as precursors of hormones known as prostaglandins. These are believed to inhibit formation of blood clots in the circulatory system and reduce blood fat levels, thereby reducing the chances of developing heart disease and strokes. Eskimos, whose diet is fairly poor and monotonous nevertheless have a very low incidence of heart disease and hardening of the arteries due to their high fish intake in general and their consumption of high doses of EPA and DHA in particular. It was shown that the blood of Eskimos did not clot as easily as that of a 'normal' westerner, taking eight minutes for a bleeding cut or wound would to clot as opposed to four minutes for the average person. It was discovered ultimately that the Eskimos intake of EPA and DHA had the effect of thinning the blood and preventing the blood from clotting. Fish oil capsules are now available in the treatment of heart and circulatory disorders in the proportion of EPA 180mg and DHA 120mg per capsule. The capsules reduce the need for the high intake of oily fish necessary to provide sufficient doses of the fatty acids. Preventative treatment requires 3 capsules daily. For the treatment of angina, hardening of the arteries, or for those who have suffered heart attacks or strokes, five capsules daily are required (1500mg EPA and DHA total). The next group of nutrients to be considered are mineral salts and these are of particular importance. From epidemiological studies it appears that some minerals have a specific action in preventing heart disease.

Magnesium

This is particularly implicated because deaths from heart disease are higher world wide in soft water areas than in hard water areas where magnesium levels tend to be high. Communities where the water supplies have been changed from hard to soft suffered increased incidences of heart disease due to losing the protective action of magnesium. In hard water more minerals are found than in soft water, the principal ones being magnesium and calcium. Calcium is also believed to exert a protective action against heart disease. In post-mortem studies those who had died from heart disease showed low levels of magnesium in the heart muscle. It is believed that magnesium dilates blood vessels in the heart, calcium having the opposite action and constricting them. A harmonious balance of both these substances ensures the healthy functioning of the heart. The best food sources of magnesium are in order of importance, soya beans, nuts, brewers yeast, wholewheat products (the refining of white flour removes 75% of the magnesium), brown rice, seafoods, dried fruits, vegetables and bananas.

Calcium

This mineral, besides combining with magnesium to protect the heart, appears to have the ability to reduce blood cholesterol levels. Low calcium levels result in high cholesterol levels. Calcium levels up to 1,200mg daily can reduce both fat and cholesterol levels possibly by combining with fatty acids to form insoluble calcium soaps which are then excreted. Best food sources are low fat dairy products, nuts beans and cereal grains. Combined calcium and magnesium supplements are available, and also dolomite which is a mineral supplement containing both these minerals.

Potassium

This removes sodium from the system which is implicated in high blood pressure. Heart attack sufferers have low levels of potassium in the heart muscles. Low potassium levels are also implicated in angina. Best sources are dried fruits, fruit and soya beans, molasses, raw vegetables, nuts, cereal grains. If salt is omitted from the diet and whole foods consumed supplements of potassium should not be necessary.

Selenium

A deficiency of this mineral causes heart disease and high blood pressure in animals and man. In epidemiological studies where the soil is low in selenium, coronary heart disease is particularly high. Where selenium intakes are high, coronary heart disease rates are at their lowest. Best sources of selenium are shellfish, wholegrain products and cereals. A supplement of selenium may be wise due to its erratic dispersal amongst the earth's soils. Absorption is more efficient from organic selenium yeast than from inorganic varieties, 250 mg daily recommended.

Chromium

This is low in the heart tissues of those dying from heart disease. It reduces cholesterol levels and may reduce the chances of developing heart failure. Sources are eggs, molasses, brewers yeast, fruit juices, wholemeal bread, cereals, wheatgerm, honey.

Manganese

Mangnese is also low in the tissues of those dying from heart troubles. Best sources - cereals, nuts, wholewheat bread, beans, fruit.

Minerals

As a general rule, in consideration of the importance of of minerals in protecting against heart disease, it may be wise to include a high quality multi-mineral in the diet which contains some of all these minerals in the right proportions. Minerals in the orotate form are the best absorbed but are quite expensive. Dolomite and kelp are excellent sources of mineral salts and are particuarly inexpensive.

Lecithin

This substance is particularly valuable in the prevention or treatment of heart disease and hardening of the arteries. It is used principally for its ability to emulsify or break down fats including cholesterol, thus preventing an accumulation of fatty deposits in the system. It contains many members of the 'B' vitamin family, particularly choline and inositol which are the main active ingredients in lecithin that are responsible for the solubilizing of fatty build ups. Lecithin is normally extracted from soya beans and is available in granule form or capsule form. In its role of reducing high blood pressure, high blood cholesterol levels and reducing blood fat, lecithin is without equal. It is used as a preventative and as a treatment for angina, heart attack, hardening of the arteries, senile dementia and Alzheimer's disease.

Vitamin E

Its main function appears to be as an anti oxidant in protecting unsaturated fatty acids from being destroyed by oxygen. Vitamin E has been found to relieve coronary thrombosis and angina due to its action in decreasing the body's need for oxygen, while at the same time increasing the supply of oxygen to the heart. It has a protective action against thrombosis and atherosclerosis. Vitamin E is an anti blood clotting agent with the ability to dissolve clots of blood already formed and the further ability to dilate (expand) the blood vessels thereby improving the circulation of the blood around the body. Vitamin E is used to treat most circulatory disorders including strokes, coronary thrombosis, atherosclerosis and varicose veins. The use of vitamin E in preventing and treating heart disease has shown exceptional results particularly under the guidance of Dr Evan Shute and his brother Dr William Shute who are the main proponents of the use of vitamin E in treating heart disease. They have used the vitamin to treat over 40,000 people in America with exceptional results. The best sources of vitamin E are wheatgerm, unprocessed vegetable oils and cereal grains.

Vitamin B6

A deficiency of this nutrient can bring about severe atherosclerosis. Foods rich in B6, including brewers yeast and wheatgerm, ought to be included in the diet.

Vitamin C

A deficiency of vitamin C can cause spontaneous breaks in capillary walls increasing the chances of a clot being formed at this point. Vitamin C has recently been implicated in the metabolism of fats including cholesterol. Evidence shows that low vitamin C levels in humans leads to higher cholesterol levels and increased fat levels in the artery walls.

Nicotinic acid (vitamin B3)

This vitamin has been shown to have a specific action in reducing high levels of cholesterol, reputedly by up to 40% in over a period of 12 weeks. This vitamin occurs as niacin but reduces cholesterol levels only in the nicotinic acid form. Whilst being extremely efficient in reducing cholesterol, this vitamin causes a flushing sensation which while being harmless is slightly uncomfortable. One 500mg tablet daily is all that is required. Natural sources are wheatgerm, liver, brewers yeast.

In conclusion, it should be clear that the solution to the problem of heart and circulatory disorders lies in observing the laws of nature and in a general constitutional effort which pays strict attention to diet. Vitamins, minerals and natural remedies will assist in breaking down fats and cholesterol, maintaining a clean, healthy bloodstream. There is no single means to prevent or treat heart disease - only a holistic effort which recognises the value of fresh air, exercise, stress control, sleep and rest and a natural diet. The adoption of these natural measures would go a long way towards rendering the scourge of heart and circulatory disorders obselete.

CHAPTER FIVE

Rheumatism and Arthritis

Arthritis and rheumatism are not terminal illnesses yet they inflict untold pain and misery on millions of sufferers. It is estimated that 34 million working days are lost annually as a result of arthritis and rheumatism and that over 8 million people seek medical help each year for treatment of these complaints.

Osteoarthritis usually affects the weight bearing joints such as the knees, hips and shoulders and is characterised by degeneration and wearing away of the smooth cartilage which acts as a cushion and shock absorber between the bones of the joint. This process of disintegration frequently exposes the underlying bone and can interfere with the membrane secretions which lubricate the joint. Calcium deposits may form around the joint causing nodules and spurs. Where calcium is lost from the spinal vertebrae the condition is known as spondylitis or spondylosis when the damage has already occurred. Arthritic degeneration in the neck is known as cervical spondylitis. Osteoarthritis can be brought on by the lack of female hormones during menopause though this complaint usually disappears once menopause is over. Lumbago is a rheumatic condition affecting the muscles of the lumbar region in the lower back, whereas sciatica is characterised by crippling pain along the length of the inflamed sciatic nerve, which runs from each hip joint to the ankle. Sciatica can either be of rheumatic origin involving inflammation of the sciatic nerve or brought about by displacement of a spinal disc vertebrae. Gout is caused by an excess of uric acid in the system usually crystallizing in the big toe and causing excruciating pain. Foods high in purine bodies, rich foods and alcohol, are implicated and should be avoided.

Rheumatoid arthritis, the most common form of arthritic complaint is characterised by inflammation of the joints, produces progressive damage and deterioration. This inflammation then proceeds to attack the synovial membranes and cartilages which eventually may become completely worn with the joint becoming swollen and distorted, losing its mobility and general function. The movement of the joint may cause grating and creaking sounds and may lose complete flexibility. The four main characteristics of rheumatoid arthritis are pain, swelling, tenderness and stiffness in the affected joint, though it can also be accompanied by loss of weight and appetite, fever and sweats, fatigue, wasting of the muscles and swollen lymph glands.

What then are the orthodox medical treatments for these arthritic conditions? Clearly they are not very successful considering the vast numbers of people suffering from these complaints. While it is possible to send man into space and destroy the world several times over with nuclear weapons it is not yet possible, in spite of the vast sums of money spent on medical research to find a cure for the treatment of rheumatic disorders. Orthodox medical treatment for arthritis and rheumatism is largely confined to the use of drugs which have a palliative and anti-inflammatory action in spite of the severity of their side-effects. Opren alone, an anti-inflammatory medicine, is believed to have been responsible for over 2,000 deaths and has now been withdrawn from the market. Aspirin is probably the most relied upon pharmaceutical remedy though this itself is implicated in damaging the stomach lining and causing internal bleeding. Surgery, however, can offer a new lease of life to the arthritic sufferer where joint destruction is beyond repair. However neither anti-inflammatory drugs nor surgery can be construed as a cure for arthritis and rheumatism. The cure is clearly to remove the cause of these ailments, allowing the body to thrive as nature intended.

Arthritis is not specifically a localised complaint affecting one particular part of the body but is, in general, a constitutional disorder of the whole system brought about by poor nutrition and a faulty lifestyle. It goes without saying that the Hunzas and other primitive societies which live in harmony with nature do not develop arthritis. It should be clear that it is the differences between their particular environment and our own which illuminate the most significant factors in the development of these diseases. The modern diet, as mentioned in earlier chapters contains an excess of animal protein and fat, an excess of concentrated starches and sugars in the form of white flour and white sugar, and an abundance of additives, chemicals, colouring agents, preservatives, pesticides, salt, coffee and alcohol. A dietary emphasis on these foods to the exclusion of fruits and vegetables, creates a build up of waste products in the system and creates a situation of internal toxaemia. It is not difficult to see that a toxic bloodstream would be a contributory factor in the onset of any arthritic condition. Fruit and vegetables are alkaline as a general rule and all other foods acid forming. Where acid forming foods are emphasised in the diet, the bloodstream will be acid and will have a corrosive action on the joints and tissue predisposing the individual towards the onset of arthritis.

That arthritis is a disorder of the whole constitution can be seen in the way that it is frequently preceded by other systemic disorders. Constipation, digestive disorders, chronic catarrh, poor circulation, varying degrees of nervous debility, fatigue and exhaustion are frequently seen in the patient before an arthritic condition develops. It has been suggested that a combination of nutritional inadequacies, excessive toxins in the system, and an excessive ingestion of modern day chemicals may cause a functional confusion of the immune system inciting its attack against the joint membranes of the body. Whatever the complexities involved in the onset and progress of arthritis several things are clear. It is of a constitutional origin and character and is amenable both to prevention and treatment through the adoption of a healthy lifestyle and a healthy diet.

The eight healing forces of nature should be observed in full involving fresh air and exercise, epsom salt baths which increase the elimination of toxic wastes, the use of gentle massage to improve the circulation, hot and cold compresses to increase the blood supply to the affected joint, and dry friction rubs with a stiff towel which again improve the circulation and the removal of waste poisons through the skin. All health building constitutional measures mentioned in earlier chapters ought to be implemented.

Diet and nutrition, however, are the most important factors in the prevention and treatment of arthritis and the following advice may prove useful. The first step is to liberate the body's own self-cleansing mechanism by adopting a largely fruit and vegetable diet. This will allow the body to remove the excess of uric acid and other waste poisons generated by a diet relying heavily on animal fats and refined carbohydrates. The pursuit of a clean, pure bloodstream fortified by the alkaline elements of fruits and vegetables should be the first goal in the prevention and treatment of arthritis. It is imperative that all devitalised foods such as white flour, white sugar, tinned and processed foods, additives, preservatives and chemical irritants be removed from the diet. Animal fats and salt should be avoided as should the excessive intake of tea, coffee and alcohol. The ideal diet would be of plant food origin involving 70% fruits and vegetables and 30% small quantities of concentrated foods i.e. nuts, seeds, beans. If animal foods are to be used then small quantities of goats milk, chicken or fish should be preferred. Sir W Arbuthnot Lane, a surgeon and authority on nutrition wrote:

'There is no longer any doubt that all forms of rheumatism are due to disturbance of the acid alkaline balance and that this condition arises from faults in nutrition. Clinical experience has now amply proved that the physical factors which predispose some people to rheumatism can only be successfully countered by a diet which puts all its emphasis upon alkaline foods'.

Natural Treatments

Acid forming foods

Meat, fish, poultry, cheese, biscuits, alcohol, spaghetti, sugar, jam, eggs, bread, all flour products, pastry, pies, soft drinks, fried foods, tea and coffee, salt, sauces, processed cereals.

Alkaline forming foods

All fruits and vegetables, with the possible exception of plums and tomatoes. Nuts, seeds, dried fruits and milk are also included in this group.

The diet should not be exclusively alkaline but should aim to correct the acid/alkaline balance. A word should be mentioned here about allergies and food sensitivities in relation to arthritis. Clinical ecologists have shown that some foods and many chemical irritants in the environment are capable of producing arthritis. Naturally the adoption of a natural diet will exclude most of these elements from the individual's environment and need not cause excessive concern.

Wheat products and cereal grains are highly acid forming, highly concentrated and difficult to digest. They are also recent additions to man's diet having been introduced only several thousand years ago, with the consequence that man is not very well adapted to their use. They contain high levels of a substance called gluten and are responsible for much mental and physical ill-health. It would be prudent to omit all cereal grains (wheat, oats, barley) and their derivatives particularly white flour products from the diet if a serious effort is to be made in combatting arthritis. Many people can tolerate cereal grains and for the individual sufferer from arthritis this must be a question of trial and error, wholegrain products only being used if well tolerated. Dr Girant Campbell in his book *A Doctors Proven New Home Cure For Arthritis'* is vehemently opposed to the use of cereal products in any shape or form in the arthritic's diet. He maintains adamantly that the adoption of a natural diet free from all canned foods, processed foods, cakes, biscuits, ice-cream, packaged cereals, bakery products, coffee, tea and soft drinks, artificial sweetners, sugar, wine and beer, certain meat products, would reduce the pain, swelling and discomfort from arthritis within a matter of weeks. He maintains that arthritis can be cured and that pain, swelling and inflammation can be eliminated completely within a relatively short period of time. He advocates abandoning tobacco, dead and devitalised bleached foods and all other chemical additives that invade man's body. The diet he advocates is little different to the natural diet already postulated in this chapter, fresh fruit and vegetables, nuts and seeds, fish and low fat fowl products. Fruits and vegetables should be eaten raw or lightly cooked but all food must be fresh. Cereal grains and all flour products are strictly taboo and must be avoided indefinitely.

Dairy products, again, are a recent addition to man's diet and should be considered as a possible allergen to the arthritic. If tolerated then low fat skimmed milk, cottage cheese and yoghurt are the superior forms and can be used in moderation. The choice foods which would comprise the best diet for the arthritic may seem spartan and unappetizing but this is not the case. It is largely conditioning and habit that drives us towards the emotional gratification of refined junk foods. Once a natural diet has been adopted for several months it is unlikely that anyone would want to return to a meat and two veg. diet. It is merely a question of breaking old habits with determination and motivation. The arthritis diet is not a special diet, it is a diet for life on natural foods which will maintain a healthy bloodstream fully nourished with proteins, vitamins and minerals. It is a diet which will slow down the ageing process to its natural pace, reduce the risk of developing major disease and instil in the individual vitality and optimism - as well as alleviating arthritis.

Cheerfulness of disposition and a positive attitude can influence the neuro-endocrine system and its internal secretions and boost the action of the immune system. Adopting a philosophical attitude and developing calmness and inner poise may help to alleviate the stresses and strains of modern life. Sleep and rest are essential to maintain the vitality of the nervous system and exercise to motivate the body's rhythms and circulation. Any measures at all which can build up the general health of the constitution and ensure the proper functioning of all the internal organs will help the individual to counteract the ravages of arthritis and rheumatism. Certain food supplements and herbal remedies are particularly useful in boosting the health of the individual against arthritis and these are as follows:

Vitamin C

It has been suggested that rheumatism and arthritis are not degenerative diseases but arise mainly from malnutrition particularly a shortage of vitamin C. Deficiencies of vitamin C in animals over a prolonged period resulted in severe impairment of the joints typical of rheumatism and arthritis. Take 2-3 grams vitamin C daily.

Vitamin B complex

These vitamins are essential to healthy nerves and protect them from the ravages of an acid bloodstream. They have a pronounced beneficial effect in cases of rheumatism.

Vitamin E

This vitamin has been very successful in experimental treatments of rheumatism with pain symptoms being vastly reduced with increased mobility of joints. Vitamin E improves the whole circulation and thus assists the regeneration of inflamed joints.

Calcium

This mineral is essential in the prevention of osteoporosis, a condition which is characterised by crumbling of the spinal vertebrae. A supplement of calcium tablets is strongly recommended both as a preventative and as a treatment. Calcium supplementation should also be used as a preventative of osteoarthritis and particularly during the child bearing years of the mother when calcium is required by the child. This will prevent osteoarthritis in later life. Calcium supplements should contain vitamin D which assists its absorption.

Cod Liver Oil

This is an important supplement in the treatment of arthritis as it lubricates the joints and provides vitamin D which aids the absorption of calcium. It provides polyunsaturated fatty acids which are believed to exert a positive influence against arthritis and to correct any dietary deficiency of fatty acids. Cod liver oil contains high levels of vitamin A which has a protective action against infection and also two particular fatty acids EPA and DHA which are precursors of hormones in the body called prostaglandins believed to possess anti-inflammatory properties.

New Zealand Green Lipped Mussell showed a striking success in trials carried out to measure its effectiveness in alleviating arthritis. Clinical trials showed 70% of rheumatoid arthritis sufferers and 40% of osteoarthritis gained varying degrees of pain relief. This particular remedy is high in mineral salts and contains anti-inflammatory properties.

Pantothenic acid (calcium pantothenate)

Commonly known as vitamin B5 this is perhaps the most important of the nutritional remedies. It is believed that there is a widespread and serious deficiency of this nutrient in the modern diet making a significant contribution towards the onset of arthritis in the western world. When rats were deprived of this vitamin they developed inflammation of the joints and other arthritic symptoms. When blood-tested all arthritic patients were found to have low levels of this vitamin, the lower the level the more serious the arthritic condition. Many scientific trials have been conducted involving high doses of this vitamin (2,000mg daily 4x500mg tablets) over periods of 3-4 months. Arthritic patients were found to have a reduction in the severity of their inflammation and a lower degree of disability and pain. The main beneficiaries of this treatment were sufferers from rheumatoid arthritis rather than osteoarthritis - vitamin B5 appears to stimulate the adrenal glands to produce anti-stress hormones and natural cortisones which appear to have an anti-inflammatory action.

Oil of Evening Primrose

This plant oil has been described as the most important discovery since vitamin C. Primrose oil contains gamma linoleic acid (GLA) and is found in substantial amounts in only one other food, mother's milk. GLA stimulates the body's production of prostaglandins which have been found to be very useful in treating a number of auto-immune diseases, rheumatoid arthritis in particular. These prostaglandins contain anti-inflammatory elements and are important in the formation of collagen. In experimental trials, two thirds of all subjects with mild to moderate rheumatoid arthritis experienced complete relief with primrose oil capsules in their daily diet. A worsening of the condition was noticed during the first two weeks followed by rapid relief.

Selenium

In Norwegian studies it was found that selenium levels were low in rheumatoid arthritis sufferers. Supplementation improved their condition markedly. Similarly sufferers from osteoarthritis experienced reduction in pain especially when combined with other anti-oxidants vitamin A, vitamin C and vitamin E. Other remedies include DLPA (DL Phenylalanine), an amino acid which reduces the destructive action of the body's own pain killers, endorphins, and thus assists in the reduction and lessening of pain to tolerable levels. African devils claw is a plant remedy which acts as a cleansing agent removing impurities from the body and acid wastes. Other herbal remedies used are Burdock, Yarrow, Elder Flowers, Poke Root, Prickly Ash Bark and Senna principally for their cleansing action and removal of uric acid from the system.

Finally, it is worth noting a comment by Dr Howard Hay on this subject:

'There is no such thing as an incurable case of arthritis, although damage done to the joints previously by years of arthritis may never be fully corrected. The process however can be halted and a great deal of improvement enjoyed in every case. There are salts such as urates (any salt of uric acid) that are actually outside the circulation deposited in the free joint cavity and not usually absorbable and so constituting a permanent crippling to just this extent. I would not touch starch or sugar in any form, but would live entirely on cooked vegetables, raw vegetables, salads, fresh fruit and milk and cheese. In addition I would suggest that you get a preparation of wheatgerm and take a tablespoon of this three times a day with honey'.

Again, the solution to the problem of rheumatism and arthritis lies in recognising and observing the laws of nature and in a concerted effort to build up the health of the whole constitution using natural forces, nutritional remedies and the healing forces of nature. There can be no single cure for arthritic disorders. Only the removal of basic causes and a return to the principles of natural health can remove the scourge of this disease from our midst.

CHAPTER SIX

Stress and Nervous Disorders

When one considers the nature of modern life and the condition of the modern technological environment, it is hardly surprising that the mental and spiritual health of an individual should be seriously threatened. When one takes into consideration the pollution of the atmosphere with lead, petro-chemicals and industrial emissions, the debilitating consequences of refined and processed foods, the frenetic pace of life, tedious and stressful work situations, shift work, night work, noise pollution, alcohol abuse, the destructive use of drugs, the upward spiralling of violence and crime, and the general emotional traumas of life which inflict themselves upon people, be it bereavement, rejection, loneliness, sickness and pain, or a combination of these and more, it is certain that the human spirit requires all the fortitude and resilience it can muster to survive in the face of such adversity.

What is more, such problems of life are likely to remain with us. In fact, considering the nature of modern society and the moral and spiritual decline in which we find ourselves embroiled, it seems likely that the problems and traumas which confront both humanity and the individual will escalate rather than subside. In the face of such adverse conditions the individual must recognise that, if it is not possible to change the world around us, it is yet possible to change ourselves and our position in the modern world. By strengthening the constitution and developing the inner self and consciousness the individual can develop considerable resilience and fortitude against the 'slings and arrows of outrageous fortune' improving the quality of life and making his stresses and strains more tolerable. To elucidate this point we should consider the nature of stress and its effect upon the individual's physical and emotional condition.

There are large numbers of people in society who from a position of mental stability and emotional normality become afflicted by a strong sense of mental ill-health out of proportion to the emotional problems that confront them. They complain of fatigue, anxiety, fear, self-doubt, loss of confidence and general inability to cope. The standard medical diagnosis is that they are suffering from some form of mental or emotional instability for which they are frequently prescribed tranquilisers, sleeping pills and anti-depressants. However this frequently is not the correct diagnosis. Just as positive and vibrant health invariably induce a sense of emotional well-being, positivity and dynamism in the individual, the converse is also true. An exhausted and debilitated physical condition will invariably induce a negative emotional state, a condition which will tend to demonstrate all forms of negative emotion, whether it be paranoia, anxiety, apathy, loss of confidence or motivation or depression.

This is an irrefutable and binding law of nature. If a condition of high energy breeds positive thought with a sense of well-being and a sense of the joy of life, then it would clearly be an admirable goal for the individual to attempt to acquire an abundance of this energy. So what is this energy? Food certainly provides blood-sugar energy and the elements and nutrients for bodily repair but a heavy meal after a tiring day will not imbue anyone with a sense of energy. On the contrary it is likely to induce sleep. Vitality is then an energy force separate from that provided by food. It is the life-force itself, a mysterious energy bestowed is us by mother nature which is restored by rest and sleep alone. This vital force flows through the nervous system and motivates every action, thought and desire. If the force of this vitality is depleted through overwork, stress, poor diet and inadequate nutrition, lack of exercise and fresh air, lack of sleep and rest, alcohol or drug abuse, emotional trauma, worry, accident or surgery, or through a combination of any of these factors and more, then individuals will experience a relative degree of fatigue and exhaustion, brought about by enervation of the vitality of the nervous system and thus a corresponding deterioration in their emotional condition.

The point is this, and must be emphasised; the condition of the nervous system and the degree of its vitality will determine to a large extent the individual's emotional condition. If the life force has been dissipated and the nervous vitality impaired there will be a corresponding degree of emotional disharmony and negativity. Any negative emotion that can be thought of will become prominent in a person's life in a condition of nervous exhaustion. These may include fear, anxiety, nervousness, timidity, irritability, loss of confidence, paranoia, apathy, pessimism, exaggeration and distortion of life's worries, claustrophobia, agoraphobia and a general sense of being under persistent and unmitigating stress. The individual will often suffer from a lack of concentration, fraught nerves, tension and a general inability to cope with life with small chores demanding extreme effort. Unfortunately too many people suffering from the above symptoms feel that they are suffering from a vague and indefinable form of mental illness. Though there is no pain from nervous exhaustion it has been described as something far worse than pain. There is a sense of overwhelming stress in a strait jacket of exhaustion where every action and activity requires excessive will-power. This condition of loss of vitality, dissipation of life force or plain nervous exhaustion is itself the greatest stress imaginable.

Far from being weak-minded or emotionally unstable the sufferer from nervous exhaustion requires tremendous strength of character and will-power to survive the unremitting stress and anguish caused by this complaint. It is this loss of nervous vitality which creates the greatest stress of all and which often makes the largest contribution to any mental breakdown which may occur. Emotional factors may well be present to a greater or lesser extent in the life of the individual sufferer but in most cases of mental breakdown, nervous exhaustion is likely to play a supporting or a leading role.

There is no demonstrable pain to nervous exhaustion, its symptoms manifesting themselves only in the spiritual condition of the sufferer. Any emotional turmoil manifested by the individual should not be confused as the illness itself but recognised as only a symptom of the real cause, the underlying nervous debility. At this point a truly vicious circle often appears, where the enervation experienced by the individual creates its own negative emotions such as fear and anxiety which in turn further deplete the life-force. This of course intensifies the severity of the anxiety and when worry and sleeplessness complete the picture, the vicious circle has been formed and the scene is set for a severe nervous breakdown. Psychiatric treatment seems not to recognise the underlying constitutional causes of much emotional illness and treats these cases with tranquilisers, anti-depressants, sleeping pills and shock treatment. It is clearly not possible to rehabilitate the individual using these measures. Sleep, relaxation and rest are the only forces which can re-charge the vitality and life-force of the nervous system and if combined with an observance of the eight healing forces of nature recovery, though exceedingly slow, can be complete. The individual ought to recognise that the causes of their debility can frequently be traced back over the preceding period, often over several years, and it is commonly found that constant stress, overwork and a degree of self neglect are in evidence. The first step to recovery is that the individual must understand the nature and causes of their debility in order to extricate themselves from the vicious circle which arises in cases of nervous exhaustion.

It is not possible to recharge the system in any other way and any aggressive efforts are doomed to failure. A long period of rest and recovery implementing the power of the eight healing forces of nature will be needed, but the individual can approach the task in the firm recognition that the body is self-rejuvenating and capable of rebuilding lost nervous energy and effecting a complete recovery. The diet is of particular importance and should emphasise natural plant foods, particularly fruits and vegetables which feed potassium and other nutrients to the nervous system excluding reliance upon meat products and refined carbohydrates (white flour products and sugar), drugs, alcohol and tobacco.

The best nerve tonic foods are brewers yeast, blackstrap molasses and wheat-germ. Supplements should include a high quality multi-vitamins and minerals containing all eleven members of the B vitamin group (Cantamega 2000 are the best produced by Larkhall Laboratories) which are responsible for maintaining the health of the nervous system. Mega nutrient therapy would be useful involving the use of moderate doses of vitamin C, vitamin E and zinc and high doses of vitamin B5 (calcium pantothenate) up to 1500mg daily to rebuild exhausted adrenal glands. Herbs are available both as sedatives and nerve tonics, including valerian root, scullcap, gentian, passiflora, hops and lupulus. Chamomile has a sedative action and is available as a tea. Fresh air and exercise in moderation should not be over-looked and an aim should be made to remain as positive and cheerful as circumstances will allow.

Meals should be light, as food makes a demand on the vitality of the nervous system in the process of digestion and assimilation. It should be mentioned here that there are factors other than nervous exhaustion which can be responsible for inducing fatigue and debility and it would be wise to consult a registered practitioner in order to eliminate this possibility before embarking upon self-treatment.

Finally it must be emphasised that recovery from nervous exhaustion is painstakingly slow and may take months and years, rather than days and weeks, depending upon the severity and degree of enervation present. The sufferer can rest assured that through judicious observance of the healing forces of nature progress will be certain and hastened to its maximum pace. In considering the subject of stress it can be safely maintained that it is invariably an inevitable aspect of the human condition. The individual's response to stress does, however, appear to be the important factor. The person suffering from nervous exhaustion experiences a distinct exaggeration of life's worries from which it is almost impossible to be extricated. Little troubles become large looming oppressive traumas, leaving the individual powerless to prevent this magnification of ills. The nervous system is frayed and exposed to the ravages of the outside world, noise at one time at acceptable levels is now of an oppressive volume, normal tasks and events which might once have been enjoyed now become irritating obstacles and chores. The behaviour of others which would once have been pleasurable, now becomes irksome and disturbing. The world in general takes on a gloomy menacing distorted appearance with the sufferer now prone to bad-temperdness, chronic irritability and irrational behaviour. It should be clear from this that the important factor in any consideration of stress is the quality of the individual's resistance. This resistance can only be maintained by preserving the vitality of one's nervous system and general health and this in itself is dependant upon removing enervating factors from one's lifestyle and observing the natural laws of health. As the vitality of the nervous system decreases the quality of life also decreases, with a certain predisposition towards negative emotion becoming inevitable. The converse is also true that in a condition of high vitality, positive emotions will be released and greater sense of the joy of life being experienced. This vitality is the first line of defence against the stresses and strains of the modern world and should be preserved and protected at all costs.

It has been shown by Dr Hans Selye of Montreal University that the body reacts to stress of all kinds in a similar way, whether the stress be in the form of accident, viruses, surgery, burns, poisoning with toxic substances, working to exhaustion, exposure to loud noises or extremes of heat and cold, exposure to X-rays or starvation.

When stress occurs the pituitary gland begins to secrete protective hormones which are carried via the bloodstream to the adrenal glands which in turn secrete chemical messengers which prepare the body to meet the stress or emergency. If the stress is prolonged or very severe then exhaustion of the adrenal glands is likely to occur to a greater or lesser extent depending on the quality of the individual's diet and intake of nutrients which provide the raw materials for building and fortifying the body's resistance. Experimental stress has shown that during periods of emergency, the body's need for all nutrients escalates.

Pantothenic acid (vitamin B5) is particularly important as an inadequacy of it prevents the adrenal glands from carrying out their normal functions of producing cortisone and anti-stress hormones. Adrenal exhaustion can be induced in volunteers through a deficiency in the diet of pantothenic acid characterised by emotional distress and bad-temperedness, severe fatigue and exhaustion, sleepiness, continuous infections, low blood pressure and muscular weakness. Within four weeks all volunteers became seriously ill. The symptoms they experienced were all typical of adrenal exhaustion and were corrected only with improved nutrition and high doses of pantothenic acid in the form of calcium pantothenate at levels up to 4,000mg daily. It would be wise for a person subjected to stress or suffering from the consequences of prolonged stress to increase their intake of nutrients through the adoption of a natural diet of wholesome foods and to increase their intake of certain nutrients including B complex, vitamin C and E and especially to take high doses of vitamin B5 (pantothenic acid) in doses of up to 2,000mg daily for a period of several months depending upon the degree and severity of the adrenal exhaustion.

There seems little doubt that due to the politics of the age, modern day materialism and the oppressive nature of the environment that incidences of stress related disorders and nervous exhaustion are likely to escalate throughout the decade of the nineties. As stress is a part of everyday life in the modern world it is clearly important to remain as strong and healthy as possible in order to be better able to cope with adversity. In a position where the individual's nervous vitality or life-force is bankrupted or where adrenal exhaustion has occurred it will no longer be possible to cope with even the most menial of tasks.

Through observance of the laws of nature with a diet that provides a high intake of nutrients, it is possible to maintain a degree of health and vigour which can absorb many of the harsh effects of stress. If sufficient attention is paid to relaxation, whether through meditation, yoga or other forms of self-awareness, then the life-force can be protected further from reckless dissipation and can be maintained in a vital condition, allowing individuals to be better able to cope with the world around them.

CHAPTER SEVEN

Common Ailments and

Natural Treatments

In this chapter a brief consideration is given to some common ailments and their herbal and nutritional treatments. Homeopathic medicines and other forms of alternative medicine are not included. It must be stated that it is always wise to consult a registered medical practitioner before embarking on a course of self-treatment, particularly in cases of severe illness. In the treatment of common ailments and disease the important factor is always to release the body's self-healing powers to remove the cause of ill-health from the individual's lifestyle.

Proper health can only be maintained and restored through observing and applying the eight healing forces of nature, as explained in an earlier chapter. Herbal and nutritional remedies are used for their therapeutic action in supporting and stimulating the body's own self-rejuvenating powers as well as to correct any possible nutritional deficiencies. The healing forces are of primary consideration in the treatment of the following ailments, the nutritional and herbal remedies taking a secondary role. A full explanation of the herbal and nutritional remedies, with a breakdown of their properties, applications and historical uses is given in the next three chapters. It must be stressed that the core of the treatment of these common ailments is building up one's constitution as a whole, paying particular attention to diet and the correct balance of nutrients. Nutrients work synergistically - they are more potent when taken as a combination of nutrients rather than in isolation.

Also it must be recognised that the body works as a whole and not in separate components. In considering the use all natural foods (fruits, vegetables, cereals, nuts, seeds, beans, yeast, wheatgerm, molasses, vitamins and minerals), these form part of all treatments.

Acne

A natural diet emphasising fruits and vegetables to maintain the alkalinity and cleanliness of the blood is essential. Nutritional remedies Vitamin A in beta-carotene form has shown some success. 25,000 i.us daily can be taken for several months reducing to a lower dose of 8,000 i.us daily after this period. Oil of Evening Primrose (500mg 3-4 capsules daily) increases the intake of essential fatty acids which are important in maintaining healthy skin. The GLA content of primrose oil has a beneficial effect on the endocrine system and is thus useful in pre-menstrual acne.

Vitamin B6 (50mg daily preferably in B complex form) is also useful in treating this complaint.

A zinc supplement is also useful in treating acne as it normalises hormone functions which are often disturbed at puberty. Take zinc orotate (100mg one daily).

Herbal remedies are are principally blood purifying agents: burdock sarsaparilla, blue flag root, or echinacea, available in herb, tablet or mixture form from any good herbalist or health food store.

Acidity

Increase in the intake of alkaline fruit and vegetables and reduce the intake of all other foods which as a general rule are acid forming. Cereal grains and all white flour products are particularly acid-forming, eggs also. Treatments include meadowsweet, charcoal, anissed, cinnamon, ginger, spearmint and peppermint. Combinations of herbs in mixture or tablet form are available from herbalists or health food shops.

Alcoholism/excessive use of alcohol

Alcohol increases the need for vitamin C (1,000mg-2,000mg daily).
The vitamin B family are destroyed by alcohol so it may be wise to include a quality vitamin and mineral supplement in the diet, or a high potency vitamin B complex supplement containing all eleven members of the B vitamin family. Vitamin B sources are molasses, brewers yeast, wheatgerm and liver. Oil of evening primrose has a rejuvenatesc the liver and has been used in the treatment of alcoholism.
(Dose 3-4 500mg capsules daily.)

Addiction

Whether to food, alcohol, cigarettes or drugs, withdrawal symptoms are featured to a greater or lesser extent. Mega vitamin therapy produces the best results in alleviating the severity of withdrawal symptoms. Take mega potency vitamin B complex one or two daily. Vitamin C 1000mg two or three times daily. Herbal treatments to counteract stress and include the use of valerian root, scullcap, gentian, motherwort.

Ageing

Over-eating and over-indulgence generally is implicated in hastening the ageing process. Experiments on animals have shown that those fed on subsistence levels of food and nutrients lived long lives and remained healthy and vital throughout. Those laboratory animals fed on demand became prone to disease, experienced hair loss and loss of youthful appearance and vigour and died at an early age. In order to slow down the ageing process to its natural pace, it is important to observe the healing forces of nature, with particular attention to diet. Avoid all refined and processed foods, particularly white flour products, sugar, animal fats and salt. Remove all unnecessary calories from the diet and emphasise a high intake of nutrients. A clean alkaline bloodstream maintained by a strong emphasis on fruits and vegetables, and a well nourished bloodstream maintained by a choice of natural foods is the magic recipe. A high quality vitamin and mineral supplement can be recommended particularly for older people whose absorption of nutrients can be impaired.
A special mention should be made here about oxygen and free radicals which are implicated in cell destruction and ageing in particular. Although oxygen is essential to life it has a corrosive quality which can be witnessed in the rusting of metals and in the way it can cause the rapid deterioration of food. Free radicals have been described as chemical agents operating within the body which have a destructive, corrosive influence upon the body's cells, causing deterioration and premature ageing. These free radicals can be formed naturally as a result of normal metabolic processes or formed as a result of environmental factors, such as the ingestion of hydrogenated fats or rancid oils, or by the inhalation of industrial chemicals and polluted air. Robert Erdmann Phd comments "At a cellular level, age degeneration appears to be largely the result of damage caused by highly reactive chemical compounds called free radicals ... Most age researchers now agree that if you can protect your body from free radicals and oxidation damage you will dramatically slow down the rate at which you age".
Fortunately there are certain nutrients which can protect the body from the destructive action of free radical agents and these are known as anti-oxidants. These are vitamin A (beta carotene), vitamin C, selenium and vitamin E. Robert Erdmann continues, "Free radical damage appears to be the very foundation of ageing ... using the anti-oxidants, researchers have been able to

significantly extend the life of animals, prevent or postpone degenerative illnesses and slow down ageing." The anti-oxidants of vitamin A (beta carotene), vitamin C, selenium and vitamin E and the enzyme S.O.D. (super oxide dismutase) work better when combined with a healthly diet of natural foods, providing all the body's nutritional requirements and are more biologically active when taken together rather than in isolation. A complete profile of each of these nutrients with recommended doses is given in the next chapter.

Allergies

In alternative medicine, the allergen is not so much the important factor as the quality of the body's resistance to the allergen. In a world oozing with chemical pollutants and irritants it is impossible to remove all potential allergens from the immediate environment. Again it is impossible to change the world around us, only ourselves and our fortitude and resilience within it. To build up the immune system all of Nature's laws should be observed with inclusion in the diet of high doses of vitamin C (3x1000mg daily), zinc orotate (100mg daily) and selenium (200mcg daily). These nutrients act as anti-oxidants against the ravages of pollution and have a specific action in building up the immune system. The single best remedy for the allergy sufferer is high doses of vitamin C, which is a natural anti-histamine, between 3-4 grams daily. A herbal remedy used is echinacea, in tablet or herb form.

The major five food allergens are wheat, eggs, milk and their by products, tea and coffee, and alcohol and should be avoided if they cause allergic reactions. Pantothenic acid (vitamin B5) is also a useful supplement as it builds up the adrenal glands which produce cortisone, a substance known to have a protective action against allergens. Hay-fever sufferers, when given cortisone before exposure to pollen, did not develop any symptoms of their ailment. The introduction of pantothenic acid into the diet can bring relief not only to hay-fever sufferers but to those allergic to house dust and other external irritants. Doses up to 2000mg of pantothenic acid in the form of calcium pantothenate should be taken daily for a protracted period as the adrenal glands do not recover from a pantothenic acid deficiency until faulty nutrition is improved. It is clearly important to fortify the whole system with sound nutrition and other health building measures if the individual is to build up a resistance to allergens. After all, most people, in spite of inhabiting a contaminated world, do not develop allergic symptoms or reactions due to the protective quality and resilience of their immune system.

Anaemia

Characterised by tiredness, palpitations and lack of stamina, iron deficient anaemia can be treated with foods rich in organic iron, particularly blackstrap molasses and brewers yeast. Iron supplements are best in the form of ferrous gluconate rather than the ferric form as it does not destroy vitamin E. All health building measures should be observed, with particular attention to nutrition, if the health of the bloodstream (haemoglobin iron levels in particular) are to be maintained. Pernicious anaemia is treatable with **vitamin B12** injections.

Angina

A nutritious diet is essential in order to break down fatty cholesterol levels, replacing saturated animal fats with unsaturated vegetable oils (oil of evening primrose or sunflower oil, for example) and increasing nutrient levels with intakes of brewers yeast, vitamin C 1-2 gram daily, vitamin E 800 i.us daily and lecithin, which assists the breakdown of fat and cholesterol.

Anorexia Nervosa

A deficiency of zinc, caused by restricted diets, can impair the individual's taste and smell, rendering food unappetising and unpalatable. The best nutritional remedy for the anorexic patient is zinc orotate (100mg one or two tablets daily). The condition is psycological in origin and appropriate steps should be taken through a medical practitioner.

61

Arthritis

All health building measures with particular emphasis on a high nutrient diet are essential (see previous chapter).

Arteriosclerosis (hardening of the arteries)

A nutritious diet low in animal fats and high in nutrients is essential. Nutritional treatments are lecithin (15-20 gram daily), vitamin E (800 i.us), vitamin C (3 gram daily), vitamin A (8,000 i.us daily). Essential fatty acids (primrose oil, sunflower oil) and fish oils can also be used in the prevention and treatment of arteriosclerosis.

Rheumatoid arthritis

Best remedies are pantothenic acid (vitamin B5) in high doses (1500mg daily - 3x500mg tablets) taken for up to six months. This is the most successful remedy in reducing inflammation due to it's action in maintaining the health of the adrenal glands which are responsible for the production of natural cortisones and anti-stress hormones. Oil of evening primrose is also beneficial to sufferers from rheumatoid arthritis due, also, to its therapeutic anti-inflammatory action. Tests have been carried out in Scotland with encouraging results showing that oil of evening primrose stimulates the body's production of prostaglandins which, in rheumatoid arthritis, are often deficient and unbalanced. Two to four 500mg capsules should be taken daily for a period of several months. This treatment can be maintained indefinitely, primrose oil being a food rather than a medicine. *Felmore Health Publications* states:

"There is a particular prostaglandin of the E type PGE$_1$, that has been found to be particularly useful in the treatment of a number of auto-immune diseases, including rheumatoid arthritis. PGE1 has prevented arthritis in rats and auto-immune disease in mice. It is an anti-inflammatory agent and reduces the release of inflammation causing lysosomes at the joints. It is also important for collagen formation. In about two thirds of all subjects with mild to moderate rheumatoid arthritis daily primrose oil capsules seemed to stop the disease process completely. Almost all those who were involved felt worse for about two weeks after beginning the therapy and then improved."

Osteo-arthritis

This disease is characterised by the gradual erosion and degeneration of the joints, with calcium outgrowths becoming prominent. Treatment is a wholesome natural diet and an intake of calcium which has been lost from the joint. Though the reasons are not well understood, calcium supplementation (between 1000mg and 1500mg daily) may cause the calcium outgrowths seen in osteo-arthritis to disappear. Calcium requires vitamin D for its absorption and this vitamin should be included in any calcium supplement taken. A natural wholesome diet, fortified with important nutrients and including adequate intakes of calcium, would appear to be the best preventative and the best treatment for also osteo-arthritis. Other natural remedies for arthritis include: devils claw, green lipped mussel extract, cod liver oil, vitamin C and herbal formulas which remove excessive uric acid from the system. Feverfew, a common plant in this country, is probably the most successful herbal remedy in the treatment of osteo-arthritis. See next chapter under Feverfew.

Anxiety

Refer to the chapter on stress and nervous disorders earlier in the book. Vitamin B complex is a natural tonic to the nervous system. Herbal medicines, including the use of valerian, scullcap, gentian, vervain are used for their sedative and calming action and also for their tonic properties in cases of nervous exhaustion. Chamomile is used as an infusion in cases of sleeplessness. Emphasis must be on strengthening the nervous system and constitution in order that life's problems can be coped with more successfully.

Asthma

A natural diet and adherence to the laws of nature in order to build up the immune system and the constitution in general are essential in cases of asthma. Vitamin C is found in abnormally small amounts in the blood of persons suffering both from allergies and asthma and can be used to relieve both conditions. When vitamin C was given to patients during asthma attacks, relief was experienced almost instantaneously in some cases and the rest within a short period of time. Attacks of asthma were also prevented when 3,000 milligrams (3 gram) of vitamin C were taken daily. This dose can be increased. Vitamin B6 (100mg taken twice daily) has proved effective also in lessening the severity of asthma attacks in both adults and children. For children with difficulty in swallowing tablets vitamin C is available in powder form and can be mixed in fruit juices. Several grams of vitamin C can be safely taken by both adults and children without side-effects. Herbal treatments include the use of Balm of Gilead, Elecampagne root, skunk cabbage, Horehound, Lungwort, Pleurisy root and Lobelia.

Back ache

If due to spinal disc troubles consult an osteopath. Pain can sometimes be relieved by vitamin C (3,000mg daily). Back ache from rheumatic pain can be alleviated by the use of herbal formulae containing burdock root, clivers, ura ursi, agrimony, poke root and elder flowers which assist the body in removing uric acid from the system and act as a general tonic to the kidneys.

Bad breath (halitosis)

Can be caused by a deficiency of vitamin B6. This complaint normally disappears when this nutrient is given. Take 2x100mg tablets daily.

Bedsores

Comfrey ointment. Comfrey contains allantoin which is a potent healing agent.

Bed-wetting

Urinary incontinence. Herbalists traditionally prescribe Cranesbill. Available in herb and tablet form.

Bells palsy

Valerian root. Available in herb or tablet form.

Birth defects

The importance of pre-conceptual care cannot be understated. Particular care should be taken to avoid tobacco, alcohol and other drugs. One cause of birth defects is a shortage of B vitamins. Lack of pantothenic acid (vitamin B5) can cause still and premature births, malformed babies and mentally retarded infants. A deficiency of riboflavin (vitamin B2) can cause congenital malformation, including cleft palate. A folic acid deficiency is implicated in neural tube defects, leading to spina bifida. Folic acid also builds up the resistance to infections in new born children. A natural diet of wholesome foods should be followed, avoiding processed and refined foods which have had their B vitamin content removed. Wholewheat cereals in particular should be avoided. It is safely recommended that a high quality multi-vitamin and mineral supplement, containing all eleven members of the B vitamin family, be taken. The best vitamin and mineral for the pregnant mother is Cantamega 1000, produced by Larkhall Laboratories.

Blood pressure (low)

Characterised by fatigue and lack of stamina, sensitivity to cold and heat, rapid pulse on exertion and excessive sleep requirements. Low blood pressure can be induced in people through a dietary deficiency of protein, vitamin C and vitamin B nutrients. A natural diet of wholesome foods is clearly essential in the treatment of this complaint. However, a deficiency of pantothenic acid (vitamin B5) is the nutrient most normally deficient in the diet of the sufferer from low blood pressure. A lack of vitamin B5 inhibits the activity of the adrenal glands in producing anti-stress hormones. Adrenal exhaustion induced by prolonged stress invariably accompanies low blood pressure. When vitamin B5 levels are increased, the adrenal glands become strengthened and low blood pressure levels should be increased to normal. Take pantothenic acid 500mg one x two daily (1,000mg) until condition improves.

Blood pressure (high)

A natural diet is essential, with consideration given to all the healing forces of nature. Salt should be avoided as it is implicated as a causative factor in hardening of the arteries thus increasing the degree of effort required by the heart to pump blood around the circulatory system.

Smoking can also be a key factor in raising blood pressure as it constricts the small blood vessels. Being over-weight makes the heart pump blood through several hundred extra miles of capillaries and places a general burden on the heart and circulation. Treatment involves natural diet, with a reduction in the intake of animal fats. These should be replaced by an intake of unsaturated vegetable oils (sunflower, olive, evening primrose) and adequate intakes of vitamin C, vitamin E, zinc and selenium which counteract free radicals circulating in the system.

An adequate intake of chromium should be maintained as a deficiency can lead to the development of arterial plaque deposits. Best sources of chromium are brewers yeast, molasses and wheatgerm. The following are a list of nutrients known to be helpful in reducing blood pressure and restoring cardio-vascular functions.

Vitamin C with bioflavonoids 1-2 grams daily. The dose can safely be increased.

Vitamin E 500 i.us - 800 i.us daily.

Vitamin B complex should also be considered for its ability to aid the body's blood stream. This group of vitamins is an essential requirement if the body is to break down fat and cholesterol in the system. Sources are wheatgerm, yeast, molasses and cereal grains.

Lecithin requires special mention due to its content of choline and inositol which have a specific action in emulsifying fats and cholesterol, allowing the body to convert them to energy. Extracted from soya beans, lecithin is available in granule or capsule form. Oil of evening primrose can be taken due to its action in reducing cholesterol and blood fat levels (500mg capsules 2-4 daily).

Vitamin B3 (nicotinic acid) has a specific anti-cholesterol action and can reduce high levels over a relatively short period of time. Doses up to 500mg daily can be taken, but this remedy does cause a flushing sensation which can be slightly uncomfortable. Nicotinic acid in time release form is preferable as this will alleviate some of the discomfort. Garlic is also a useful treatment in high blood pressure. Other herbs used are principally hawthorn berry, motherwort, scullcap, capsicum and passiflora.

Blood clots (thrombosis)

Known as coronary thrombosis when concerned with the heart and cerebral thrombosis (or stroke) when affecting with the brain. Treatment is vitamin E (500 i.us - 800 i.us daily) due to its anti blood-clotting activity and lecithin, because of its choline and inositol content which breaks down fat levels in the blood. Fish oil capsules containing EPA and DHA fatty acids (which act to thin the blood and prevent the formation of blood clots) may also be used - up to five 1000mg capsules daily are recommended.

Boils

Normally an indication of low zinc levels. Use zinc orotate (100mg one or two tablets daily).

Bronchitis

Responds to vitamin A in beta carotene form (25,000 i.us daily) which stimulates the mucous membrane of the respiratory tract to resist infection. Vitamin C (1000mg - 2000mg daily) increases resistance to infection. Herbal remedies are useful and include capsicum, lobelia, coltsfoot, euphorbia, liquorice, pleurisy root, senega, wild lettuce.

Bruises and swellings

Prevention of unnatural bruising requires vitamin C (1-2 grams daily) with bioflavonoids. External applications benefit from knitbone or comfrey either in leaf or ointment form.

Burns

The healing process is increased by massive doses of vitamin C and normal quantities of vitamin E (500 i.us daily). The best local applications are vitamin E cream or honey dressings.

Cancer

The alternative approach to cancer is geared towards stimulating the body's own healing powers and, in particular, to building up the individual's immune system and the vigour of its response to cancer cells.

Diet is of particular importance and emphasis should be placed on fruits, vegetables, nuts, seeds, beans and cereal grains, with animal foods and all refined and processed foods being omitted.

Supplements are used heavily in the alternative treatment of cancer. Vitamin C is used rigorously (up to 10 grams daily). Beta carotene (vitamin A) 10,000 i.us daily or obtained from carrot juice. Laetrile (vitamin B17) is used for its anti-cancer activity but requires professional treatment.

Selenium is often prescribed since epidemiological studies indicate that in areas where the soil is low in this mineral salt cancer rates tend to be high. The converse is also true, high selenium areas have low incidences of cancer. Animal experiments have indicated that some cancers can be cured with selenium supplementation, due to its action in invigorating the immune system and toughening the cell membrane rendering it more resistant to attack from cancer causing antigens. As a preventative 100mcg of selenium daily is recommended, preferably in the form of selenium yeast which increases its absorption in the body.

Bromelain, a digestive enzyme extracted from pineapple, is used for its ability to de-shield the protein coating of the cancer cell, rendering it more vulnerable to attack from the body's immune system. A complete guide to supplements and alternative therapies used in cancer treatment is given in an earlier chapter.

Finally, as always, professional advice should be sought in the treatment of cancer rather than embarking on a course of self-treatment.

Candida Albicans

This is the name given to a yeast which exists within all of us and which is normally confined by the body's own immune defence mechanism. The over extensive use of antibiotics, a diet excessive in sugar and refined carbohydrates and use of the contraceptive pill can weaken the individual's immune system making one more susceptable to the disease. Symptoms include depression, anxiety, stomach disorders, heartburn, allergies, migraine, fatigue, bloatedness, cystitis, menstrual problems, thrush, irritability and pre-menstrual tension. Treatment is by natural diet, excluding all sugary and yeast foods on which the candida organism thrives. For the special diet consult *Candida Albicans* by Leon Chaitow (Thorsons Publishing Group).

Treatment also includes the use of nutritional supplements which build up the health of the immune system. These are;

Vitamin C (1000mg x 3 daily).

Vitamin B complex mega potency.
(Two daily. Must be yeast free).
Selenium (200mcg daily).
Zinc orotate (100mg one daily).
Vitamin E (500 i.us one daily).
Beta carotene (25,000 i.us daily).
Oil of evening primrose (500mg 2-4 daily).
A specific remedy is available in the treatment of candida, and this is an extract from coconut oil named caprylic acid which has a noted anti-fungal action. This remedy is available in capsule form as Capricin.

Cataracts

Can be caused by a deficiency of vitamin B2 (riboflavin). Use whole B complex, one or two tablets daily. Vitamin C 1000mg, two daily. Calcium (500mg daily) also can be taken.

Catarrh

Often caused by a build up of waste products in the system, generated by the excessive consumption of concentrated foods i.e. fats, proteins and carbohydrates. Dairy products, in particular milk, cheese, butter and eggs, are especially mucous forming. When the body's organs of elimination (the bowels, lungs, kidneys and skin) are over run by toxic poisons and waste products, the body uses the mucous membranes as a safety mechanism for the removal of this excess build up of catarrh. The discharge of mucous is to be encouraged rather than suppressed.
A diet emphasising the clean, watery foods of fruits and vegetables and a drastic reduction in the consumption of concentrated starchy, protein and fatty foods will provide the best results in eliminating catarrh. Herbal medicines which invigorate the body's own self-cleansing mechanism are available in the treatment of this complaint including the following plants: vervain, sage, boneset, lobelia, raspberry, quassia, echinacea and garlic. Vitamin C 2000mg daily and zinc orotate 100mg daily are used to strengthen the immune system against infection and allergy.

Chillblains

Can be treated with nicotinic acid (vitamin B3) which dilates the capillary arteries, thus improving the blood supply to the affected part. 500mg daily. Rutin, a biflavonoid, has historically been used in circulatory disorders due to its action in maintaining the elasticity of blood vessels and capillary arteries. Rutin (3x60mg tablets) can be taken daily. This bioflavonoid acts in a similar way when used for other circulatory disorders, including haemorrhoids and varicose veins.

Cholesterol

This is a fatty substance with important functions in the body. It exists as either HDL (high density lipoprotein) cholesterol or LDL (low density lipoprotein) cholesterol. A high ratio of HDL to LDL is required to protect against arteriosclerosis and coronary heart disease. HDLs are increased by taking unsaturated fatty acids, either from food sources or from oil of evening primrose (2000mg daily) and vitamin E (500 i.us daily). High blood cholesterol levels can be reduced by taking 2000mg vitamin C daily.
Recent information indicates that the use of nicotinic acid (vitamin B3) has a specific and dynamic action in reducing cholesterol levels. Doses up to 500mg daily. Lecithin granules can also be incorporated into any effort towards reducing cholesterol levels, due to its action in emulsifying fats.

Circulation (poor)

Remedies used to improve the circulation are as follows:
Vitamin E (500 i.us daily) due to its action in dilating the blood vessels and its anti-blood clotting properties.
Peppermint oil which has a tonic and stimulant action.
Rutin which dilates the capillary arteries thereby increasing the circulation and blood supply (60mg tablets are available). Take one three times daily.
Nicotinic acid (One 500mg tablet daily).

Cirrhosis of the liver

Vitamin B complex to overcome multiple deficiencies of vitamins and minerals, particularly B vitamins which are destroyed by alcohol.

Oil of evening primrose (500mg 4 capsules daily). This remedy has a rejuvenating and toning action on the liver.

A high quality vitamin and mineral may be useful to counteract multiple nutrient deficiencies.

Claudication (intermittent)

Pain in the calf muscles due to narrowing of the blood vessels.

Treatment is with vitamin E(500 i.us once or twice daily).

Rutin (60mg one three times daily).

Peppermint oil capsules (one three times daily).

Colds

Take 1000mg of vitamin C every four hours until relief is obtained. Recent discoveries show that zinc gluconate in lozenge form (providing 25mg of zinc gluconate per tablet) relieved the symptoms within 24 hours and with 80% relief within five days. This remedy only works if the zinc is sucked as this liberates the zinc to infiltrate the mucous membranes where it exercises its antibiotic properties.

Zinc does not work in the treatment of colds if swallowed whole though it does have a toning action on the immune system. In the treatment of colds, take ten zinc gluconate lozenges 25mg daily for three days, when symptoms should subside. Garlic is also a natural preventative.

Cold sores

May be prevented or treated with zinc supplements. Take zinc orotate (100mg once or twice daily). Vitamin C (2000mg daily) and zinc applications are also useful.

Colitis

Fasting under medical supervision is the best treatment for the sufferer of ulcerative colitis. This allows the body the best opportunity to heal the inflamed and ulcerated colon. Once healing has taken place a natural diet fortified with additional vitamins and minerals, including yoghurt to replace the intestinal flora, should maintain the health of the colon.

Constipation

All plant foods contain fibre, but animal foods and refined cereals (white flour products) contain none at all. Herbs can be used to assist the functions of the bowels and formulae including cascara, dandellion root, myrrh, fennel and holy thistle are available from herbalists or health food shops. Senna pods are noted for their laxative properties, with the plant being infused and the liquid drunk. Bran can be added to the diet, though there ought to be sufficient fibre in a diet of natural foods to render this unnecessary.

Coughs

Herbs used include liquorice, aniseed, ipecacuahna, coltsfoot, horehound, hyssop, skunk cabbage and elecampagne root. As a preventative, the immune system can be fortified with vitamin C (1-2 grams daily). Garlic is also a natural preventative.

Contraceptives

Oral contraceptives increase the body's requirements for certain vitamins:

Vitamin B complex (containing 50mg B6, folic acid and B12)

Vitamin E (200 i.us daily).

Vitamin C (1000mg daily). Take at a different time from the pill.

Convalenscence

A high quality vitamin and mineral plus vitamin C, up to three grams daily, will enhance recovery.

Cramp

Treat nocturnal cramp with vitamin (E 500 i.us) before bedtime plus vitamin C (1-2 grams) daily.

Cysts (breast)

Vitamin E (500 i.us) daily.
Oil of evening primrose six 500mg capsules daily.

Cystitis

If related to proliferation of the candida albicans yeast, the anti-fungal remedy of capricin (caprylic acid) is recommended. Herbal remedies used in the treatment of cystitis confine themselves principally to the use of buchu leaves. Cranberry juice is also a beneficial natural remedy and is available in liquid or capsule form.

Dandruff

Vitamin B6 deficiencies result in scaliness of the skin and excessive dandruff. Treat with mega potency vitamin B complex containing 50mg B6 until symptoms subside. Include yeast and wheatgerm in the diet.

Depression

Can be induced through shortage of B vitamins, particularly vitamin B6. Treat with mega potency vitamin B complex. Depression can be either a physical or emotional state. If physical, use the eight healing forces of nature to restore health using, mega vitamin therapy. Vigorous health and vitality will help the individual to cope with the inevitable traumas and stresses of life. If the depression is related to hormone difficulties, oil of evening primrose capsules contain GLA which stimulates the body's production of oestrogen.
Take four 500mg capsules daily, along with a mega potency vitamin B complex. Korean ginseng and vitamin E are also useful in boosting the body's levels of vitality.

Dermatitis

Can be caused by a lack of vitamin B complex, beta carotene (vitamin A) or essential fatty acids. Treat with high potency B complex once or twice daily.
Beta carotene (25,000 i.us daily).
Oil of evening primrose (500mg 4-6 capsules daily).
Zinc orotate (100mg one daily) can also be useful.

Diabetes

Consult a registered practitioner. Periwinkle herb (vinca major) can be useful in reducing high blood sugar levels. Vitamin E is highly recommended due to its action in improving the circulation.

Diarrhoea

Can be caused by a deficiency of vitamin B3 and may respond to supplementation with whole B complex.
Herbal medicines are available from herbalists or health food stores.

Digestive tract

Gastric ulcers can be prevented by high doses of vitamin E 500 i.us daily.
Treatment of gastric ulcers respond to high doses of beta carotene (up to 150,000 i.us daily for five weeks). There is some indication that vitamin
It is believed that supplementation may prevent stomach cancer, 10,000 i.us daily being the normal dose recommended. There are a number of plants used for their healing properties, including golden seal root, comfrey root, marshmallow root and cranesbill root.

Duodenal irritation

Some herbs and plants contain potent healing properties and are frequently used by herbalists in the treatment of these conditions. The plants used include principally the following: comfrey marshmallow root, cranesbill root and golden seal root.

Dry skin

Treatment with beta carotene 25,000 i.us daily and oil of evening primrose 500mg (4-6 capsules daily). Vitamin E cream can be used externally.

Eczema

This condition should be treated by attempting to build up the constitution as a whole through strict observance of nature's eight healing forces.

Particular attention should be paid to the diet avoiding all refined and processed foods, sugar and animal fats.

Dairy products are strongly implicated as a causative factor in eczema, the problem often arising in infancy with the child developing an allergic reaction to the introduction of cow's milk into the diet. Cow's milk and its by products of cheese and butter should be omitted from the diet for several months to see if progress occurs. Goats milk can safely be substituted. Eczema can be caused by a deficiency of essential fatty acids in the diet normally provided by plant oils, particularly a deficiency of G.L.A. (gamma linoleic acid) which is found in evening primrose oil. Take primrose oil capsules (500mg 3-6 capsules daily). Eczema has also been induced in volunteers through a lack of B vitamins in the diet. Take a mega potency B complex supplement twice daily and include brewers yeast, molasses and wheatgerm in the diet. Zinc orotate 100mg one or two daily can also be effective particularly if combined with vitamin C (1000mg 2 or 3 tablets daily). Progress can be slow and should be persevered with for 4-6 months. Infantile eczema normally responds to treatment with G.L.A. from primrose oil capsules (4-6 capsules daily). The oil can be squeezed onto food from the capsule. Other treatments for eczema include the use of beta carotene (25,000 i.us daily).

Eye-sight

Dependant on adequate vitamin A. Take a beta carotene supplement or include carrot juice in the diet. Itching under the eyelids and bloodshot eyes can be a symptom of vitamin B2 deficiency. Heavy smoking disturbs vitamin B12 levels which can lead to impaired vision. Take whole B complex one or two daily.

Fatigue

Many possible causes. If brought about by overwork, stress or anxiety then nervous exhaustion must be considered. Treatment is with sleep and rest. A deficiency of vitamins and minerals may be implicated and this can be corrected through dietary improvements and mega vitamin therapy. Whatever the cause of fatigue, due consideration must be given to all the healing forces of nature with emphasis placed on removing the cause from the individual's lifestyle.

Gall stones

Tests showed that animals given a diet deficient in vitamin E all developed gall stones, though no stones occurred in animals receiving the vitamin. It is generally believed that diets high in cholesterol and saturated fat are the main causes of gall stones though animals fed large amounts of these foods showed no signs of developing stones as long as the vitamin E intake is adequate. Vitamin E (500 i.us daily) is recommended as a preventative.

Gingivitis (inflammation of the gums)

High doses of vitamin A required in beta carotene form (50,000 i.us daily for 4-6 weeks).Also vitamin E 500 i.us daily and vitamin C (2-3 grams daily).

Glandular fever

Treatment is with mega vitamin therapy including a mega potency B complex and vitamin C (2000-3000mgs daily).

Glaucoma

Adequate intakes of beta carotene and B vitamins particularly riboflavin (B2) should be emphasised. Pressure behind the eye ball may be reduced by taking vitamin C (2-3 grams daily).

Gout

Caused by uric acid crystals which settle in toe and finger joints. Treatment with natural diet reducing the intake of rich concentrated foods. Red meat or fruit can aggravate the condition. Plants used by herbalists are principally for their action in removing uric acid from the system; blue flag root, capsicum, guaia gum resin and uva ursi.

Haemorrhoids

Can be caused by constipation thus implicating diet as a causative factor. Rutin is a successful treatment. Take 600mg daily in tablets of 60mg strength. Ointments are frequently used containing Pilewort and Witch Hazel.

Hay fever

Treatment is geared towards fortifying the individual's immune system and it's response to external allergens. Treatment is with high doses of vitamin B complex plus additional pantothenic acid (1000mg daily) in order to build up the adrenal glands and their production of anti-stress hormones. Vitamin C is also effective in high doses 3-4,000mg daily, due to its anti-histamine action.

Heart disease

Nutrients used in prevention and treatment are as follows:
Vitamin B complex (one daily)
Vitamin C (1-2,000mg daily)
Vitamin E (500 i.us daily)
Saturated fats (animal fats) should be replaced by unsaturated fatty acids, sunflower oil, safflower oil, olive oil, primrose oil. If primrose oil is used (take 3-4 capsules daily).
Fish oils contain EPA and DHA fatty acids which are precursors of prostaglandins known to inhibit the development of blood clots and reduce blood fat levels. Take two or three 1000mg capsules daily.
Minerals are implicated in the health of the heart, particularly calcium, magnesium and selenium. A natural diet should provide most of these minerals, though if living in a soft water area a magnesium/calcium supplement is recommended to correct the deficiency of these minerals. Selenium is required in only small amounts though due to its exceptional importance in the prevention of both heart disease and cancer and its poor distribution amongst the earth's soils it may be wise to take a selenium supplement, (approximately 200mcg daily) preferably in the form of organic yeast selenium.
Chromium is a mineral which appears to be beneficial in preventing heart disease through its action in controlling cholesterol levels. High quality multi-minerals supplements are available which contain all the minerals mentioned and are available in orotate form for maximum absorption.

Hepatitis

Can be relieved by high doses of vitamin C if caused by viral infection.

Hiatus hernia

Plants used by herbalists for their healing properties include golden seal root, marshmallow root, comfrey root and cranesbill root.

Hyperactivity

Remove all artificial additives and colourings from the diet. Success has been gained through the use of vitamin C (1000mg daily) and oil of evening primrose (500mg 2-4 daily), due to their action in bolstering the body's defence mechanism, thereby lessening the action of allergens.

Impotence

The important factor is to attempt to purify the bloodstream of waste products and toxins through the adoption of a natural diet emphasising principally fruits and vegetables.

A pure, clean, alkaline bloodstream fortified by vitamins, minerals, enzymes and other nutrients is the only lasting cure for this complaint. Vitamin A (25,000 i.us daily) in beta carotene form is essential for the body's production of sex hormones. A zinc deficiency can cause reduced sexual function. Take zinc orotate 100mg one or two daily reducing intake to one tablet after two months. Zinc is also believed to stimulate the body's production of testosterone. Plants used by herbalists in the treatment of this complaint include Saw Palmetto berries, Mexican Damiana leaves and Kola nut. Special emphasis is placed on Korean ginseng for its ability to increase the body's production of natural steroids.

Incontinence

Treatment by herbalists usually with cranesbill root.

Infertility

Causes can be complex and deep rooted, but for milder cases treat with vitamin E (500 i.us daily).

Insomnia

Herbalists normally use valerian root for its sedative properties. Camomile and passiflora have a milder sedative action. Tryptophane is an amino acid traditionally used in the treatment of nervous disorders and sleeplessness.

Kidney stones

Treatment with vitamin B6 (100mg) preferably in vitam in B complex form plus magnesium (300mg daily). The action of these nutrients is to suppress kidney stone formation by dissolving calcium and its deposits from which most kidney stones are formed. Herbalists recommend buchu leaves made into an infusion for those with a tendency to form kidney stones.

Leg ulcers

Best results have been obtained with zinc orotate supplements 100mg taken three times daily for two months reducing to one daily, and the application of zinc ointments. Vitamin E is also beneficial in improving the circulation and blood supply. Herbal ointments are available containing caster oil and witch hazel.

Liver problems

Diseases of the liver can cause a loss of the vitamins stored there, particularly vitamin B complex. Oil of evening primrose is believed to have a regenerating effect on the liver (4x500mg capsules daily). Clearly a natural diet and the avoidance of alcohol is an important consideration in the treatment of liver problems.

Lumbago

Treatment with 4x500mg tablets of pantothenic acid daily for 3-4 months.

Memory (poor)

Can be corrected by thiamine, available in B complex form. Lecithin granules are useful due to their choline content which maintains the health of the nervous system.

Menière's disease

Characterised by ringing in the ears, deafness and vertigo. Treatment is with members of the B vitamin family, thiamine and riboflavin, preferably in the form of vitamin B complex. Nicotinic acid can also be taken individually up to 500mg daily reducing the dose gradually to that which maintains relief.

Menopause

Known as the change of life, this is a period when menstruation ceases. This is frequently characterised by emotional and physical symptoms of ill-health including headaches, hot flushes, putting on weight, depression, irritability, rapid mood changes, self-pity and frustration. Some emotional problems associated with the menopause may be alleviated by positive thought, but the major approach of natural medicine relies on revitalising the general constitution and invigorating the workings of the endocrine system and its output of hormones.

During menopause the woman's glandular system undergoes a major transformation with the body's production of oestrogen diminishing gradually, bringing about emotional and physical upheaval.

Hormone Replacement Therapy (HRT) frequently administers doses of oestrogen to combat the diminishing levels of this hormone in the body, though this treatment is not without side-effects and rarely provides the panacea of good health that is wished for. Superior results have been gained with the use of vitamin E which not only appears to normalise the body's levels of oestrogen but also improves the heat-regulating mechanism of the body. It also normalises levels of sex hormones and dilates the body's blood vessels thus improving the whole circulation. Approx 600 i.us vitamin E daily ought to be taken to be effective.

Ginseng is another remedy which has been discovered to have a remarkable action in boosting the body's production of hormones and thus alleviating the distress of menopausal symptoms. The chemical structure of ginseng resembles that of the body's sex hormones and anti-stress hormones has a therapeutic action in boosting the body's production of oestrogen.

Studies have been done to confirm the benefits of ginseng. 72 volunteers received ginseng and some vitamins whilst a further 72 ladies received only placebos. Of the 72 receiving ginseng 43 reported that symptoms of hot flushes and night sweats disappeared whilst in the placebo group little success of any description was reported. It is estimated that four out of five women experiencing problems in the menopause can expect a marked improvement from taking ginseng root.

In further trials approximately 80% of volunteers who were suffering from a range of menopausal complaints experienced dramatic improvements in their condition. Korean ginseng is the best form of ginseng available and can be provided by 600mg tablets. One or two tablets daily is all that is required.

No discussion of herbal treatments in the menopause would be complete without mention of oil of evening primrose. It has been discovered to contain a substance that is found in high concentrations only in mother's milk. This substance is known as gamma linoleic acid (GLA for short) and it is this essential fatty acid which imparts to oil of evening primrose its miraculous properties.

Oil of evening primrose and more specifically GLA, stimulates the body's production of hormone-like substances known as prostaglandins which act as the body's regulators and messengers and which are involved in the growth and regeneration of the body cells, regulation of the blood pressure and significantly in maintaining the health of the endocrine system. Oil of evening primrose is of particular value in the menopause as it appears to regulate the body's production of oestrogen and exerts a beneficial action in reducing the severity of menopausal symptoms including hot sweats, fatigue and irritability.

A deficiency of essential fatty acids can cause poor skin tone and lifeless complexion, eczema, hair-loss, poor resistance to infection, painful swollen joints, liver damage, lethargy and fatigue and may inhibit the body's absorption of calcium. For these reasons it may seem wise to include primrose oil as a nutritional supplement in the diet, particularly during the menopause and other times of menstrual discomfort, in order to take advantage of its fatty acid profile. For more information on oil of evening primrose see the glossary on herbal and nutritional remedies in the next chapter. For use during the menopause, between 1000mg and 3000mg of primrose oil can be taken daily, preferably in the form of 500mg capsules 2-6 daily.

The importance of a healthy diet during the menopause cannot be stressed too highly and a a strong effort should be made to include only natural, wholesome foods in the diet. The eight healing forces of nature should be observed in full, paying attention to the importance of exercise which maintains the health of the bones and exerts a beneficial influence in the prevention of osteoporotic disease. See osteoporosis.

Mega vitamin therapy may prove beneficial during the menopause with particular emphasis being given to vitamin B complex which can alleviate many of the nervous disorders experienced during this time and also to calcium, which aside from its value in maintaining the health of the nervous system, is of paramount importance in strengthening the bones and preventing osteoporosis. Calcium is often undersupplied in the Western diet but is of particular importance during the menopause as falling levels of oestrogen during this period tend to reduce the body's ability to absorb and utilise calcium. Any supplements of calcium should include vitamin D which assists the body to absorb this important mineral.

Iodine is important in preventing underactivity of the thyroid gland which can cause loss of vitality, depression, loss of sexual desire and increase in weight. The best sources of iodine are seafood and kelp tablets.

The use of wheatgerm, brewers yeast and blackstrap molasses can also be recommended during this period due to their high concentrations of vitamins, minerals, trace elements and organic iron. Whilst a strong effort should be made during the menopause to strengthen the constitution as a whole and to bring the body to a state of health and harmony, sufficient attention should be given to the power of positive thought in improving the quality of life and in its capacity to stimulate and invigorate the neuro-endocrine system and its internal workings and hormonal secretions.

Menstruation

Most problems associated with pre-menstrual tension such as irritability, depression, fatigue, bloatedness, headaches, nervousness and mood swings can be reduced through a diet of natural foods and judicious supplementation with certain vitamins, minerals and herbal medicines. Dr Guy Abraham, a pioneer in the field of PMT states that "PMT is a very real and very regular form of suffering for many women. It has an effect that goes well beyond mere physical discomfort. It affects the way a woman functions in her job, in school, or at home with children and husband. It can cause marital strife and even lead to divorce. But with attention to diet and proper nutrition a woman can relieve the symptoms and even eliminate them altogether".

The first step is to cut out refined sugar as it depletes the body's reserves of B vitamins and magnesium, nutrients which have a specific role in the prevention of menstrual problems.

Dairy products should be reduced in the diet preferring low fat varieties, and animal fats reduced drastically. Caffeine should be avoided because it aggravates some symptoms of PMT particularly tenderness and swelling of the breasts. This means cutting out not only coffee, but chocolate, some fizzy drinks and tea in excess. An excessive salt intake should also be avoided as this can cause water retention and bloatedness. As a general rule cut out sugar, white flour products, caffeine, chocolate, processed and refined foods, and cut down drastically on salt, meat products, dairy products and alcohol. Include in the diet fruits, vegetables, cereal grains, nuts, seeds and beans.

Certain nutritional supplements can be used in the treatment of PMT. Vitamin B6 (pyridoxine) assists in the metabolism of oestrogen and in the normal functioning of the pituitary gland. It is used to alleviate symptoms of PMT including aggression, nervous tension and. irritability. Optimum levels of vitamin B6 are approximately 150mgs daily with 50mgs of this amount being provided by a vitamin B complex supplement, the other 100mgs provided by a traditional B6 100mg supplement.

All members of the B vitamin family are important in the treatment of PMT because they assist the liver in its function of breaking down excess oestrogen. Foods rich in B vitamins, such as molasses, yeast and wheatgerm, should also be included in the diet along with any B complex and B6 supplements.

The mineral magnesium has been found to be of particular benefit to sufferers from PMT. When the hormone oestrogen builds up in the blood stream it has an irritant effect on the nervous system, producing symptoms of nervousness, irritability and fatigue. The liver has the task of breaking down the body's levels of oestrogen but cannot perform its functions adequately without B vitamins and vitamin B6. Neither the liver nor the B vitamins however can perform their duties without adequate levels of magnesium in the body. Magnesium is found in green vegetables, wholegrains, brown rice and particularly nuts and seeds. Magnesium supplements can be obtained with one 500mg tablet daily being the recommended dose, preferably in orotate form. If magnesium orotate 500mg tablets are not available or are considered too expensive, then high potency dolomite tablets can be preferred which contain both magnesium and calcium, two or three tablets daily being all that is required.

Vitamin E has been shown to be effective in reducing tenderness of the breasts in 85% of women and in reducing most general symptoms of pre-menstrual tension. Vitamin E is an anti oxidant and protects the adrenal and sex hormones from being destroyed by oxygen.

Oil of evening primrose is probably the best known and most successful remedy in the treatment of PMT as it contains gamma linoleic acid, an essential fatty acid which stimulates the body's production of prostaglandins. It is believed that an imbalance of prostaglandins, particularly low levels of prostaglandin PGE1, are a significant factor in pre-menstrual tension. Capsules are available in 500mg strength two to four capsules to be taken, either daily, throughout the monthly cycle or ten days prior to the period.

Migraine

This is a distressing complaint that affects large sections of the population. Clearly the best approach to the eradication of this ailment is to discover the cause of the migraine and to remove it from the individual's lifestyle. This is not particularly easy considering the vast numbers of chemical pollutants which exist in the air and water and the large numbers of additives, pesticides and preservatives that contaminate our food. Alternatively, the migraine trigger may be related to stress or the work environment, which may not be particularly easy to modify. However, much can be done to ease the plight of the migraine sufferer.

The naturopathic view of migraines is that they are merely a symptom of an underlying disordered state of the system, and that the pain experienced is only an indication of physical disharmony rather than the illness itself. The body is composed of millions of cells whose role in life is to receive nutrients and expel the waste products. These cells are surrounded by fluids from which they receive their nutrients. When these extra cellular fluids become burdened with toxic wastes, whether due to over consumption of concentrated foods or a lowered vitality of the system, the body itself initiates a migraine attack in order to relieve the pressure in the inter cellular fluids and to allow the body the opportunity for cleansing toxic wastes from the system.

It is noticeable that during migraine attacks a compulsory fast is imposed, making the intake of food impossible until the system has had time to recover. Migraine may well be nature's own way of initiating the healing power of fasting in an effort to restore bodily equilibrium and harmony. It follows from this that if internal toxaemia is a predisposing factor in migraine then the factors which cause this toxaemia should be removed from the individual's lifestyle.

An excessive consumption of concentrated foods i.e. fats, proteins and carbohydrates should be avoided preferring instead the cleansing foods of fruits and vegetables. All concentrated foods generate waste products in the system which need to be removed by the organs of elimination. The foods which generate the most toxic by-products are animal foods, meat products in particular, dairy products, refined white flour products and white sugar.

A natural diet of fruits and vegetables, nuts, seeds, beans and cereal grains, with the avoidance of additives and preservatives, junk foods, salt, alcohol and coffee should go a long way towards reducing the levels of migraine in our society. Migraine should be looked on as a constitutional disorder, brought about by general disharmony of the system. All efforts at building up the general constitution should be made with rigorous observance of the healing laws of nature. Vitamin and mineral therapy is frequently useful with particular emphasis being placed on high doses of members of the B vitamin family. One high potency B complex should be taken twice daily. Extra calcium pantothanate (vitamin B5) can be taken 500mg daily. Magnesium has been shown to alleviate migraine in certain people 500mg daily required preferably in the form of magnesium orotate.

Allergens would appear to make a significant contribution towards levels of migraine and the individual will need to experiment with exclusion diets in order to ascertain any offending elements. If the cause of migraine cannot be discovered or removed from the individual's environment then the herbal remedy feverfew is available which has shown truly spectacular results in tests.

Feverfew, known as the aspirin of the 18th Century, was used for pain relief in headaches and toothache, women's problems, stomach disturbances and fevers. In clinical trials carried out at the City of London Migraine Clinic, successful results were obtained in over 70% of sufferers.

The evidence of feverfew's success is largely gained from testimonial evidence by the thousands of people who have benefited from use of the plant, rather than from scientific analysis. It has however been discovered that feverfew contains a group of substances known as sesquiterpene lactones, the most important of which appears to be parthenolide. Much scientific investigation has yet to be carried out on the feverfew plant though its success appears to result from its action as an anti-inflammatory agent, its ability to regulate the body's production of prostaglandins and its influence in inhibiting platelet aggregation (the clumping together of the body's platelets in the blood stream).

For more information see under Feverfew in the next chapter. In the treatment of migraine one 200mg feverfew tablet is all that is required daily, one tablet being the equivalent of four fresh leaves. The plant can be eaten in its natural state though it is very bitter and acrid to taste. The remedy should be taken for a minimum period of three months before full benefit can be expected. In some people feverfew can cause mouth ulcers and should be discontinued. Feverfew should not be taken during pregnancy.

Mouth ulcers

These normally result from a deficiency of zinc in the diet. Successful prevention and treatment has occurred with zinc supplementation preferably zinc orotate 100mg one or two tablets daily).

Sore lips and cracks at the corners of the mouth are normally caused by a deficiency of B vitamins or linoleic acid (occurring in plant oils particularly primrose oil), whereas a sore mouth and tongue nearly always implicates a deficiency of B vitamins.

Muscular Dystrophy

Some success with vitamin E, preferably taken with selenium.

Multiple Sclerosis

A strictly natural diet excluding dairy products and cereal grains has been known to show marked improvement and prevent deterioration. Mercury leaking into the bloodstream from dental fillings (amalgam) has been implicated as a possible causative factor. Oil of evening primrose is a useful treatment as it maintains the myelin sheath that covers the nerves and spinal cord. Two to four 500mg capsules should be taken daily.

ME (Myalgic Encephalomyelitis)

This is an illness known as Post Viral Fatigue Syndrome or, in the United States, Chronic Fatigue and Immune Dysfunction Syndrome. ME is often preceded by a common viral infection with flu like symptoms from which the victim does not recover quickly.

Symptoms include severe muscular fatigue which is worsened by exercise, causing, headaches, dizziness, loss of concentration, short term memory, nausea and aching joints.

Depression and emotional problems are a feature of ME but these are a symptom not the cause. ME may be precipitated by viral attack though it appears likely that the problem lies principally with the individual's immune system and its inability to overcome particular viruses. Treatment then is constitutional in origin, with all attempts being directed towards building up the strength of the immune system. It is important to avoid any elements in the environment which may deplete the vital force of the immune system such as common allergens, food additives and preservatives and any toxic pollutants that contaminate air, food and water.

Mega nutrient therapy is specifically recommended, emphasising the anti-oxidants vitamin A, C and E, with high doses of vitamin C being particularly important due to its anti-viral properties. Beta carotene and zinc are also particularly important in maintaining the healthy functioning of the immune system. Pantothenic acid may be useful due to it's action in maintaining the health of the adrenal glands, which can be exhausted during prolonged stress.

Osteoporosis

This condition mainly affects women at the menopausal or post menopausal stage of life, due to decreasing levels of oestrogen, (a hormone which is important in the assimilation of calcium from the bloodstream). Osteoporosis is characterised by thinning and crumbling of the bones, principally the spinal vertebrae, the thigh bone and the shorter arm bone, and is usually progressive, causing much pain and distress. Grace J Harstad in an article on osteoporosis writes, "There is no question that lowered oestrogen levels lead to bone loss".

At menopause, the decline of oestrogen from the ovaries alters the secretion of hormones from other glands in the body. As a result the cells responsible for breaking down bone become more active than those that build bone. Osteoporosis usually shows up 10 to 20 years after natural menopause, or within 4 to 11 years if a woman has her ovaries removed before that time. The earlier menopause occurs the more likely a woman is to develop osteoporosis.

Women who smoke reach menopause an average of five years earlier than non-smokers and bone loss after menopause occurs 50% faster amongst smokers. Excessive coffee drinking also leads to increased bone loss as this interfiers with calcium absorption. A high protein diet also leads to bone degeneration. A diet containing 95 grams of protein per day will cause a daily calcium loss of 26mg. Vegetarians who eat eggs and dairy products have much healthier bones than meat-eaters.

In the prevention of osteoporosis sufficient attention ought to be given to the importance of exercise in creating the muscular contractions and tensions which are essential for proper bone development.

Other preventative treatments for osteoporosis include the use of wholesome natural foods including fruits and vegetables, nuts, beans, seeds and cereal grains with inclusion of calcium rich low fat dairy products.

It is estimated that after the age of 35 a woman needs 1200mg to 1400mg of calcium daily with only an average of 600-800mg daily being provided by the modern diet. A natural diet will increase the calcium intake but supplements of this mineral ought to be strongly considered (between 500mg and 1000mg daily).

Calcium supplements should always include vitamin D which is essential for the absorption of this essential mineral (approximately 800 i.us daily). Calcium supplements are available which provide 250mg of calcium with 400 i.us of vitamin D per tablet. Two to four tablets daily would provide a sound insurance against calcium deficiency in general and osteoporosis in particular. Vitamin C should also be taken daily as this vitamin is required for the formation of cartilage and connective tissue, which maintains the strength and resilience of the bone structure.

Vitamin C is recommended in doses of 1-2 grams daily. Essential fatty acids are also required for the proper absorption of calcium and these can be provided by plant oils, sunflower, safflower or olive oil or oil of evening primrose capsules.

Osteomalacia

A condition where the bones have softened due to lack of vitamin D, causing low levels of calcium.

A high calcium intake is required with extra vitamin D supplied by cod liver oil.

Pernicious anaemia

Symptoms are fatigue, weight loss and loss of appetite.

Treatment is with vitamin B12 injections, admistered by prescription and continue throughout life.

Phlebitis

This condition is caused by a blood clot or thrombosis in a leg vein. Prevention is with 400 i.us - 500 i.us vitamin E daily. Treatment with a slightly higher dose (up to 800 i.us daily). Professional medical advice should be obtained for this condition.

Prostate troubles

Enlargement of the prostate gland is a common male complaint affecting a large section of the population, particularly in old age. Fatty acids high in cholesterol increase the individual's chances of prostate inflammation. Reducing dietary fat and cholesterol appears to reduce the size and swelling of an inflamed prostate.

Prostatitis, causing acute pain and discomfort, has been treated successfully with zinc supplements in orotate form. Men with chronic prostatitis normally have low zinc levels in their prostate gland and semen. Low zinc levels have also been found in patients with cancer of the prostate. A natural diet of wholesome natural foods, with a reduction in the intake of animal fats, is essential in the prevention and treatment of prostate troubles.

Nutritional supplements should include a high quality vitamin and mineral and zinc orotate tablets of 200mg daily for a period of several months when the dosage can be reduced. Pumpkin seeds are particularly high in zinc and should be included in the diet. Lecithin supplements in capsule or granule form should be taken in order to break down blood cholesterol levels. The most outstanding results however in the treatment of enlarged prostate glands has been with oil of evening primrose. James Hart and William Cooper MD of Los Angeles carried out experiments on sufferers from inflammation of the prostate gland and concluded that primrose oil was largely curative of this complaint. An experiment involving 19 patients was conducted using only oil of evening primrose as a treatment; with the following results;

1) All cases showed a lessening of residual urine.

2) For 13 of the 19 patients the treatment ended their having to get up during the night to urinate.

3) There was a decrease in fatigue and leg pains and an increase in sexual libido in all cases.

4) Cystitis, or inflammation of the bladder, cleared up as the residual urine disappeared.

5) Dribbling was eliminated in 18 of the 19 cases.

6) The force of the urinary stream was increased.

7) In all cases the size of the prostate gland rapidly reduced.

Oil of evening primrose capsules (500mg strength 4-6 daily) were used throughout the trial.

Psoriasis

Characterized by dry, scaly skin due to the excessive production of epithelial cells. Treatment should emphasise a mainly fruit and vegetable diet, including nuts, seeds and beans and wholegrain cereals. Coal tar and cortisone ointments may burn off the top layer of affected skin but cannot be considered a cure. A period of fasting on a restricted diet of fruits, vegetables and their juices is a particularly good way of alkalising the bloodstream and removing toxic poisons from the system. Psoriasis has been linked with having excessive amounts of cholesterol in their bloodstream. Extremely successful results have been found when lecithin granules (up to 8 tablespoons daily) have been given to psoriasis sufferers in order to break down the body's fat and cholesterol levels. (It should be remembered that lecithin (see next chapter) contains choline and inositol, two B vitamins, with the specific action of emulsifying and breaking down fats in order that the body can use them as energy.

A deficiency of essential fatty acids can also contribute to the development of psoriasis and can be corrected with one or two tablespoons of cold pressed sunflower oil, safflower oil or oil of evening primrose capsules (500mg up to 6 daily). It is also widely considered that psoriasis can result from faulty utilisation of fats with sufferers having excessive amounts of cholesterol in their bloodstream. Extremely successful results have been found when lecithin granules (up to 8 tablespoons daily) have been given to psoriasis sufferers in order to break down the body's fat and cholesterol levels. (It should be remembered that lecithin (see next chapter) contains choline and inositol, two B vitamins, with the specific action of emulsifying and breaking down fats in order that the body can use them as energy). The best regime for the psoriasis sufferer would be as follows:

Avoid all refined and processed foods, additives and preservatives, animal foods and animal fats, cows' milk, cheese, eggs, white flour products, sugar, salt, citrus fruits, red wine and excess alcohol, spicy, smoked and pickled foods. Tobacco should also be avoided. A natural diet should be observed emphasising fruits and vegetables and all other natural foods, nuts, seeds, beans and cereal grains. In the initial stages supplements should be heavily included in the dietary regime in order to ensure efficient absorption of fat and cholesterol and to stimulate the body's own healing powers.

These are: mega potency vitamin B complex. (2 or 3 tablets daily).

Oil of evening primrose capsules (500mg 4-6 daily).

Beta carotene (50,000 i.us daily).

Lecithin granules (4-6 tablespoons daily).

Zinc orotate (100mg daily).

Treatment should be continued for 4-6 months, when dramatic improvements should be experienced. Nutritious foods such as wheatgerm, brewers yeast and molasses should be included and all the healing forces of nature adhered to vigorously.

Scurvy

A disease characterised by fatigue, weakness, bleeding gums, gingivitis, loss of weight and muscular aches and pains. Treatment is with vitamin C to correct the deficiency responsible for this complaint (up to 3,000mg daily).

Senile dementia

Best results have been obtained from the use of lecithin granules or capsules due to their concentration of choline with its capacity to improve memory and some mental functions.

Shingles

A viral infection of the central nervous system causing pain in the nerve endings. High doses of vitamin C every 3 hours has relieved pain. Vitamin B complex is also useful in helping to clear nerve lesions. Herbalists traditionally prescribe Valerian Root for the treatment of this compaint.

Sexual debility

Rejuvenation of sexual vitality demands a natural diet of wholesome, nutritious foods in order to supply adequate vitamins, minerals, trace elements and enzymes. It also requires a clean alkaline bloodstream which can be gained only through a heavy reliance on fruits and vegetables in order to allow the body's organs of elimination maximum opportunity to remove toxic waste products from the system.

Specific supplements which can be useful are zinc orotate (100mg one tablet daily) which can increase blood levels of testosterone in males. Beta carotene is also an essential nutrient in the body's production of sex hormones (25,000 i.us daily being recommended). Herbal medicines traditionally used in the treatment of sexual debility include the use of saw palmetto berries, kola nut and mexican demiana leaves. Korean ginseng is particularly beneficial due to its action as a general stimulant and tonic and its ability to increase the body's production of hormones.

Sunburn

People especially prone to sunburn can increase their tolerance levels by taking high doses of para amino benzoic acid (PABA), a member of the vitamin B family. When taken daily, exposure to sunlight can be tolerated many times more than when the vitamin is not taken. All usual precautions must be taken when the sun is particularly stong, especially by the fair-skinned. PABA sun creams are also particularly effective in preventing sunburn. Night creams and moisturisers containing PABA appear to exert a beneficial action in preventing wrinkles and ageing skin. PABA is also a useful prevention of prickly heat rash. In preventing sunburn and encouraging a golden tan without burning 500-1000mg PABA should be taken daily whenever exposure to the sun is anticipated. For further information see glossary under PABA.

Stretch marks

Beneficial results in prevention and treatment have been gained with vitamin E supplementation (up to 600 i.us daily). Pantothenic acid has also shown beneficial results due to its action in stimulating the adrenal glands and their secretions of anti-stress hormones. Zinc is also a useful preventative and can be taken in orotate form at levels of (100mg daily).

Strokes - see chapter on Heart and Circulation Disorders

Prevention and treatment is with Vitamin E up to 600 i.us daily, Vitamin C 1000mg daily, oil of evening primrose 500mg 4-6 capsules daily. Lecithin, either granules or capsules, is used for its ability to dissolve and emulsify fats and cholesterol. Fish oils containing E.P.A. and D.H.A. are used for their action in thinning the blood and preventing blood clots, (3-4 1000mg capsules daily).

Stress - see earlier chapter on Stress-Nervous Disorders

The adrenal glands can be exhausted by prolonged stress and require pantothenic acid (vitamin B5) to restore them to healthy functioning (3x500mg tablets should be taken daily). The body's requirements for all the B vitamins increases in times of stress. Include brewers yeast, wheatgerm and molasses in the diet along with a high quality of vitamin B complex supplement. Vitamin C levels should also be increased in times of stress, up to 3000mg daily.

Surgery

All vitamins should be used to speed up the healing process especially vitamin C (up to 3000mg daily) and zinc orotate (100mg one or two daily). Vitamin E is also useful in assisting recovery (up to 600 i.us daily).

Travel sickness

Treatment with vitamin B6 (100mg daily) and ginger root capsules (adults 3-4 daily, children 1-2).

Tinnitus

If caused by high blood pressure then follow the treatments for this complaint. Hawthorn Berry is traditionally prescribed by herbalists under these circumstances. If the problem is caused by catarrhal deafness then treatment should include a diet emphasising fruits and vegetables and low in mucous forming dairy products. Herbal medicines are available to assist the body's cleansing effort and come highly recommended. Research has discovered a dynamic relationship between nutrition and tinnitus, and a strong effort should be made to include wholesome natural foods in the diet with the eradication of refined and processed foods. Correcting dietary inadequacies has produced considerable relief and some cures in up to 90% of sufferers.

Varicose veins - see treatment of Heart and Circulatory Disorders

A natural diet emphasising fruits and vegetables in order to maintain the cleanliness of the blood stream is essential. All of the healing forces, particularly exercise should be observed vigorously. Nutritional supplements are of great benefit in the treatment of varicose veins. Rutin, a bioflavounoid which strengthens capillary walls and dilutes blood vessels is recommended at daily intakes (between 60mg and 600mg daily). Vitamin E prevents the blood from clotting and improves the general circulation. Doses up to 800 i.us daily can be safely taken. Peppermint oil is a useful herbal remedy, reducing tiredness and aching in the legs and invigorating the whole circulatory system. Available in herb, tablet, powder or oil form.

Warts

External applications include slippery elm and thuja ointment. Internal treatments include the use of beta carotene (in high doses up to 50,000 i.us daily) taken for up to 4 months when the warts should disappear.

Water retention

Pharmaceutical water tablets (diuretics) prescribed by the doctor often remove potassium from the system, a mineral salt whose importance cannot be over-emphasised. It is more appropriate to consider the cause of water retention and to remove it from the individual's life style.
Poor nutrition and excessive intakes of salt (sodium) are the principal causes of water retention and as such strong efforts should be made to adopt a natural diet of fruits and vegetables, cereal grains, nuts, beans and seeds and to eliminate junk foods and refined and processed foods from the diet. Fruits and vegetables should form 70% of the diet due to their high potassium levels. These have the ability to take excess sodium (salt) out of the system.

Nutritional supplements can be included in the diet, emphasising vitamin C, a natural diuretic, (up to 300mg daily); vitamin B complex and oil of evening primrose (2-6 500grm capsules daily) which is a particularly good source of esential fatty acids. Other known sources of ESF's include sunflower, safflower and soy bean oils (one tablespoon daily).

Salt should be studiously avoided, along with all the foods in which it is a hidden ingredient. Salt causes water logging of the body's tissues and fluids and is the single, most important causative factor in water retention. A natural diet providing all the necessary nutrients will confer great health benefits on the individual assisting the constitution in its efforts to maintain normal fluid levels. Herbal diuretics traditionally prescribed by alternative practitioners and herbalists include the following plants: juniper berry oil, broom, parsley piert, dandelion root, clivers, uva ursi, buchu and boldo leaves.

Weight Loss

The solution to weight-loss is quite simply to observe nature's laws, adopt a diet of natural foods providing all the nutrients necessary for maintaining the body's metabolic rate and and general harmony. Take plenty of exercise and use vitamin, mineral and essential fatty acid supplements where necessary.

A simple technique for losing weight rapidly is through the adoption of a high protein diet to the exclusion of carbohydrates and fats, though this is not a natural or healthy diet and should not be adopted over long periods.

Proteins generally do not contribute much to weight gain, while carbohydrates and fats are energy foods loaded with calories. A simple milk-egg-protein powder mixed in skimmed milk and used to replace a meal is a suitable way of initiating a weight-loss programme, is vastly superior to most weight loss powders on the market, and infinitely cheaper. Carbohydrates (starches and sugars) should not be omitted from the diet as these provide the body with energy and fuel, though they should be reduced, along with fats, on a weight loss plan.

A diet of 70% fruits and vegetables and small quantities of fat, proteins and carbohydrates, will ensure that weight levels become normalised and permanent. All nutritional supplements can be used with beneficial results, including vitamin C (which acts as a natural diuretic), oil of evening primrose to provide essential fatty acids, lecithin granules or capsules to break down fat levels in the body, kelp to provide iodine which maintains the health of the thyroid gland and vitamins and minerals to act as a general normaliser of the system and metabolic tonic.

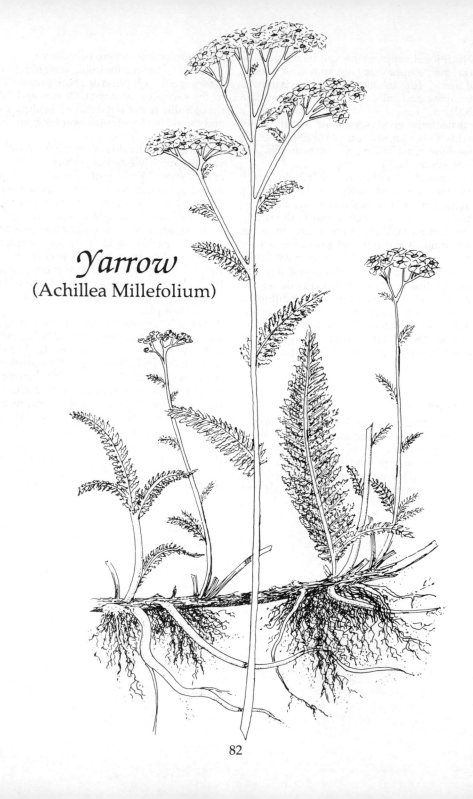

Yarrow
(Achillea Millefolium)

CHAPTER EIGHT

GLOSSARY OF NUTRITIONAL REMEDIES

VITAMIN A

Found in fish liver oils particularly cod liver oil. Occurs as beta carotene which the body converts into vitamin A in fruits and vegetables, particularly carrots, broccoli, spinach, cauliflower, cabbage, apricots etc. Fish liver oil sources of vitamin A can provide toxic amounts of this vitamin as it can be stored in the liver. Vitamin A converted in the body from beta carotene is non toxic and is the preferred form of use. Beta carotene has been found recently to exert a protective action against cancer, particularly cancers of the lung, stomach, oesophagus and cervix. Persons with low intakes and plasma levels of beta carotene were found to be more susceptible to these forms of cancer. Studies have shown that the risk of developing lung cancer, even amongst cigarette smokers is reduced considerably by high intakes of beta carotene from fruits and vegetables. Beta carotene also has a protective action against skin cancer caused by direct exposure to sunlight and is particularly valuable as a protective agent against sunburn and for people who are sensitive to sunlight. It should be used with a sunscreen agent, preferably containing PABA, a vitamin particularly effective in preventing sunburn. Beta carotene is converted into vitamin A in the human intestines and the liver though not all of it is absorbed. The beta carotene that is not absorbed enters the bloodstream where it is laid down in the fatty layers of the skin as a yellow tanning pigment. Beta carotene can be used then as a tanning agent without the sun, though obtaining sufficient sources from food alone is difficult and requires supplementation. Carrot juice is often used in alternative cancer clinics for its high levels of beta carotene, being consumed until the skin develops a golden brown hue where intakes are then reduced. Beta carotene is also useful in building up the body's resistance to infection particularly respiratory infection and in the treatment of bronchitis where it stimulates the mucous membrane of the respiratory tract to resist infection. It is used in the treatment of acne, eczema and in strengthening the immune system. Beta carotene can also shorten the duration of illness, help the removal of age spots, improve hair and skin quality, counteract night blindness and weak eye sight and can promote strong teeth, bones and gums. Beta carotene supplements are available in doses from 10,000 i.us to 25,000 i.us daily.

VITAMIN B COMPLEX

These vitamins are water soluble and so any excessive intake is excreted in the urine. They are consequently non-toxic and need to be replaced in the system daily. The B vitamins are also synergistic, ie they work together, and are more potent when combined than when taken in isolation (with some exceptions which will be mentioned later).

VITAMIN B1 (THIAMINE)

Deficiency causes fatigue, constipation, irritability, depression, lack of concentration, nausea, emotional disturbances, sciatica and neuritis. It has a beneficial action on the nervous system, enhances mental ability and can boost morale. Anyone who is a smoker, drinker, on the pill or consumes large quantities of sugar has a greater need for this vitamin. An excessive consumption of refined carbohydrates can cause a deficiency of thiamine, due to refining processes which remove this vitamin from food. Surgery, illness, pregnancy and all forms of stress can create an increased need for this vitamin. Alcohol also destroys vitamin B1 as it interferes with the vitamin's utilisation by the liver. Therapeutic uses for thiamine include the treatment of beri-beri, lack of concentration and lowered mental ability, alcoholism, lumbago and sciatica. It is also used as an insect repellant, releasing an odour through the skin pores to which insects have an aversion.

VITAMIN B2 (RIBOFLAVIN)

This vitamin (available in high quality vitamine form, mineral supplement and mega potency B complex) is yellow in colour and stains the urine similarly. A deficiency of riboflavin causes bloodshot and tired eyes, a feeling of gravel under the eyelids and a sensitivity to light, loss of hair, sores and cracks in the corner of the mouth, mouth ulcers, nerve weakness, dizziness and insomnia. Riboflavin promotes healthy skin and hair and is useful in the prevention of gastric and duodenal ulcers. This vitamin is easily destroyed by light, alcohol and tobacco. Any one taking the pill or who has a poor or restricted diet should increase their intake of this vitamin.

VITAMIN B3 (NICOTINIC ACID - available as nicotinamide or niacin)

This vitamin is essential for a healthy nervous system and for the synthesis of sex hormones. It maintains healthy skin, tongue, digestive system and brain functions. A deficiency of niacin causes pellagra characterised by dermatitis, dementia and diarrhoea, also muscular weakness, fatigue, irritability, stress and depression. Its therapeutic uses include the treatment of schizophrenia, alcoholism, tobacco addiction and high blood cholesterol levels. In the treatment of schizophrenia dramatic results were obtained when patients were given high doses of nicotinic acid (between 3gms and 6gms daily). It was suggested that schizophrenia could be a biochemical abnormality which prevented absorption of the vitamin from the bloodstream to the brain demanding higher than normal levels of nicotinic acid than could be provided by a normal diet. Alcoholics showing similar mental symptoms to schizophrenia were shown to benefit greatly from high doses of nicotinic acid in nicotinamide form - up to 6gms daily being given. Nicotinic acid can also be used to help tobacco smokers give up the habit. Nicotinic acid is also particularly successful in reducing blood cholesterol levels (nicotinamide or niacin do not have this ability). Trials done repeatedly since the 1950s indicate that cholesterol can be lowered with nicotinic acid up to 40% over a period of 8 weeks on a daily dose of 2-3grms daily.

Nicotinic acid causes the blood vessels to dilate and, in high doses, causes a flushing sensation of the face and upper body. American research suggests that excessively high doses can cause liver damage and for this reason it may be wise to take nicotinic acid tablets in time release form at 500mg strength - a level of intake which is perfectly safe.

Nicotinic acid also relieves arthritic conditions and the pain from joint degeneration but only so long as the vitamin therapy is continued.

VITAMIN B5 - (Known as pantothenic acid or more usually calcium pantothenate)

This vitamin is distributed widely in the plant food kingdom, a factor which reflects its importance as a nutrient. It is involved in the production of energy and in the metabolism of fat and cholesterol; it is important in the formation of antibodies and in the production of anti-stress hormones; it helps to maintain a healthy nervous system and assists the body in detoxifying drugs. A deficiency of pantothenic acid can cause aching, burning and throbbing of the feet, loss of appetite, respiratory infection, neuritis, arm and leg cramps, depression, insomnia, fatigue, psychosis and a lack of hormone production. Pantothenic acid is destroyed in food processing, particularly of whole grain products, but is relatively stable during cooking. This vitamin is required in higher than normal amounts after stress or injury due to its action in maintaining the health of the adrenal glands and their secretions of anti-stress hormones. Antibiotic treatment frequently destroys intestinal bacteria which are capable of synthesising pantothenic acid. Therefore additional pantothenic acid may be required to compensate for these losses. Pantothenic acid is also useful in counteracting the toxic side effects from drug medicines and antibiotics. The most important action of pantothenic acid, however, appears to be its effect on the adrenal glands in conditions of stress. This function requires some elaboration. Dr Hans Selye of Montreal University, a renowned medical scientist whose findings have been proven conclusively in thousands of scientific studies, discovered that all forms of stress, whether in the form of overwork, drastic surgery, burns, car accidents, worry and anxiety, x-rays, extremes of heat or cold, loud noises, drugs or viruses, or running on a treadmill until a point of exhaustion, affected the body in basically the same way. When stress first occurs, the pituitary gland releases protective hormones which are carried in the bloodstream to the adrenal glands which are activated to produce cortisone and other chemical messengers, which in turn activate the body to meet the emergency. When the diet is adequate and the stress not too severe or prolonged, the body is able to cope with this emergency and to maintain healthy functions. If the stress is intensive, as in major surgery or serious accident, or if it is simply prolonged, the body may arrive at a situation of pituitary and adrenal exhaustion from which a long period of rest, a nutritious diet and mega vitamin therapy (with heavy emphasis upon pantothenic acid) provides the only antidote.

Experiments have shown that rats receiving pantothenic acid swam up to four times further than those receiving no pantothenic acid. Experiments on human volunteers showed that when given pantothenic acid they were able to withstand enormous stresses without the normal consequences of protein destruction, rising blood sugar and salt retention. Furthermore volunteers fed upon an adequate diet with the exception of pantothenic acid showed a marked decrease in the levels of adrenal hormones produced by the body. They became quarrelsome, irritable and emotionally disturbed, developing low blood pressure, chronic fatigue and weakness and continuous respiratory infections. They showed all the symptoms of chronic adrenal exhaustion with levels of adrenal hormones decreasing steadily as the experiment progressed. Within 25 days all the volunteers were seriously ill and it required 4,000mg of pantothenic acid daily over a period of several weeks before the adrenal glands and their hormonal secretions were restored to normal.

Deficiencies of pantothenic acid have also been shown to lower the individual's resistance to infection, particularly respiratory infection, due to the importance of this vitamin in the production of antibodies with their specific ability to counteract invading bacteria and viruses. A deficiency of pantothenic acid is also implicated in the widespread prevalence of allergies in modern society. Children given 100mg of pantothenic acid daily showed a reduction of 50% in their allergic reactions to foreign substances. The same dose of pantothenic acid also manifested the ability to reduce coughs and stuffiness produced by excessive mucous secretions caused by an allergic response.

A deficiency of pantothenic acid has also been shown to cause arthritis and bone degeneration in experiments on animals. In humans, meat-eaters were shown to have less pantothenic acid in their bloodstream than vegetarians. The significant factor being that those suffering from arthritis had far lower levels of pantothenic acid in their system than those not suffering from the disease. In fact the lower the levels of pantothenic acid in the bloodstream the more serious were the arthritis symptoms. Tests were then conducted by Dr Barton Wright in which pantothenic acid, in the form of calcium pantothenate, was administered daily. Within seven days blood levels of pantothenic acid had risen steadily paralleled by a noticeable alleviation of the arthritis pain of the volunteers. Larger trials were then carried out with doses up to 2,000mg daily of calcium pantothenate being administered to nearly 100 patients. Results were again impressive with a noticeable reduction in swelling, stiffness, pain and disability experienced by the arthritic patient. However, success was limited to the treatment of rheumatoid arthritis, with little success being noted in cases of osteo-arthritis. It would appear that the success of pantothenic acid in the treatment of the inflammatory condition of rheumatoid arthritis is due to its ability to stimulate the adrenal glands to produce anti-stress hormones, including cortisone, which can prevent the development of the inflammatory and degenerative diseases. Pantothenic acid is completely safe and non-toxic and should be taken in calcium pantothenate form in tablet strength of 500mg. In the treatment of rheumatoid arthritis 4x500mg tablets (2,000mg daily) of calcium pantothenate can be taken daily for a period of approximately 4 months when the dose can be reduced to 1 or 2 tablets daily. Similar doses of up to 2,000mg daily can be taken in cases of severe stress, adrenal exhaustion, allergies and poor resistance to infection. The best natural source of pantothenic acid includes brewers yeast, liver, nuts, wheatgerm, soya beans, wholegrain cereals and beans. Pantothenic acid is widely distributed amongst foods though it is easily destroyed in food processing and being water soluble is frequently lost in cooking. It is also destroyed in the system by the use of antibiotics and by prolonged stress.

VITAMIN B6 (PYRIDOXINE)

This vitamin is water soluble and is involved in the metabolism of amino acids from protein. It is essential for a healthy nervous system and for normal nerve and brain functions. A lack of vitamin B6 can cause splitting of the lips, scaly skin, nervous problems including mental depression, convulsions, migraines, irritability, puffy fingers and ankles and breast discomfort. Vitamin B6 can be lost in cooking and is destroyed in milk by treatment at high temperatures. It is also destroyed by alcohol, smoking, some drugs and the contraceptive pill. The best food sources are: brewers yeast, wheatgerm, oats, soya beans, bananas, nuts, wholewheat products, brown rice, potatoes. Depression in women induced by taking the contraceptive pill can be treated with 100mg vitamin B6 daily. In the treatment of pre-menstrual problems. Doses of vitamin B6 given daily at levels of 100mg showed marked improvements particularly in removing headaches, the most common symptom in pre-menstrual tension. Deficiencies of vitamin B6 can cause arteriosclerosis, a condition where fatty plaque deposits congest the arteries reducing the passage of blood. Monkeys given a diet adequate in all nutrients except vitamin B6 rapidly developed arteriosclerosis. The condition can be reversed and fatty deposits emulsified and broken down when B6 is re-introduced into the diet. Vitamin B6 has also been used successfully in the treatment of allergies, hay fever and bronchial asthma, particularly in children at doses of 100mg daily.

Vitamin B6 is also valuable in the treatment of morning sickness and in pregnancy at doses not exceeding 25mg daily. It has a therapeutic value also in the treatment of infantile convulsions and travel sickness (at doses of 50mg to 100mg daily). Vitamin B6 can also prevent the formation of kidney stones particularly when combined with magnesium.

CHOLINE

A member of the B vitamin family but not recognised as a true vitamin. Choline is a lipotropic factor which means it is involved in breaking down fats and cholesterol and allowing the body to use them as energy. Choline prevents fatty deposits from accumulating in the liver and prevents both fats and cholesterol from being laid down in the arterial walls. Choline, due to its action in breaking down fats, plays its part in preventing and treating most diseases of the heart and circulatory system including high blood pressure, coronary thrombosis, strokes and arteriosclerosis. A lack of choline can also cause nerve degeneration, senile dementia and low resistance to disease. Natural sources of choline include liver, wheatgerm, brewers yeast, egg yolks, cereal grains, nuts and pulses. The highest natural source of choline is provided by lecithin which contains 3,430mg of choline per 100grms lecithin.

INOSITOL

A water soluble member of the B vitamin family but not a true vitamin. Inositol, like choline, is also a lipotropic agent with the ability to break down levels of fat and cholesterol in the body, thus being used in the prevention and treatment of heart and circulatory disorders. Inositol also occurs in high concentrations in the nerves of the brain and spinal cord and appears to exert a calming influence on the nervous system reducing irritability and anxiety. Inositol is also believed to be a useful treatment in baldness with it's ability to stimulate hair growth. Natural sources of inositol are as follows: liver, wheatgerm, brown rice, cereal grains, brewers yeast, nuts, molasses and pulses. Like choline, inositol is a major constituent of lecithin and occurs in high doses in lecithin granules, containing 2857mgs inositol to 100grms of lecithin. Both choline and inositol are best supplied in the diet by lecithin.

BIOTIN

Symptoms associated with biotin deficiency include fatigue, depression, nausea, sleepiness, loss of reflexes, hair loss, loss of appetite, increased cholesterol levels and muscular pain. Biotin is implicated in a wide variety of body functions including the metabolism of carbohydrates, fat, protein and unsaturated fatty acids and is consequently necessary to maintain healthy skin, hair, sweat and sex glands, and nerves. Biotin can be destroyed by the use of antibiotics, by cooking and stress. Natural sources include liver, eggs, yeast, wheatgerm and wholegrain products. Recent studies indicate that a deficiency of biotin may also be implicated as a causative factor in cot deaths.

FOLIC ACID

A water soluble member of the B vitamin family. A deficiency causes megaloblastic anaemia, characterised by fatigue, breathlessness, irritability and certain mental disturbances including sleeplessness, forgetfulness and confusion. A deficiency may also cause spina bifida and premature births. Folic acid is necessary for the metabolism of RNA and DNA nucleic acids (which are essential in transmitting hereditary characteristics) and also for building up resistance to infection in infants and babies. Folic acid can be destroyed by light and air, drugs, the contraceptive pill, excessive over cooking of foods and is often poorly absorbed from food in the elderly. Widespread deficiencies of folic acid in the modern diet have been noted amongst the population but particularly in women during the last 3 months of pregnancy. The best natural sources are brewers yeast, soya beans, wheatgerm, nuts, green leafy vegetables, wholegrain, beans, eggs and brown rice.

VITAMIN B12 (COBALAMIN)

Occurs exclusively in animal foods. A deficiency causes nerve degeneration, mental disturbances, menstrual disorders and leads to pernicious anaemia. Vitamin B12 is best administered by injection form when it is used as an appetite stimulant and to correct mental confusion, paranoia, fatigue, poor memory and mood swings. Vitamin B12 levels can be reduced by veganism, alcohol abuse, heavy smoking and old age.

PABA (Para Amino Benzoic Acid)

A member of the B vitamin family, PABA prevents the greying of hair and is essential to the growth of bacteria. It is beneficial in the treatment of vitiligo, a condition characterised by the appearance of light areas on the skin. PABA is best known as a sunscreen agent, being used both in sun creams and in supplement form to prevent sunburn. PABA in doses of 500mgs to 1000mgs daily has been shown to increase tolerance in sunlight in people prone to sunburn, allowing up to 100 times greater exposure to the sun. Richest food sources of PABA are yeast, molasses, wheatgerm, liver and eggs.

VITAMIN B17 (Laetrile)

This vitamin has been discussed thoroughly in the chapter on cancer and alternative therapies. Laetrile is used in natural treatments for cancer due to its cyanide content which is believed to exert a specific anti-cancer action, but is used only as part of a general wholistic approach. Richest natural sources are apricot and peach kernels, apple and pear pips, bitter almonds and cherry and plum stones. Laetrile is available in the treatment of cancer only on prescription if injections are required.

The vitamin B complex family clearly have a multiplicity of important functions in the body and their value cannot be overstated. They are important in maintaining a healthy nervous system and operate as the anti-stress vitamins, preventing emotional and mental disharmony and are a natural tonic and anti-depressant. They are frequently lost in the cooking of foods and can be destroyed by alcohol, sugar, some drugs, exposure to heat and light, and stress. Natural food sources always implicate wheatgerm, brewers yeast, molasses as the chief suppliers of these vitamins, though if these foods are not part of the individual's diet then a vitamin B complex supplement can be taken, particularly if large quantities of alcohol are consumed. The following eleven B vitamins should all occur in any vitamin B complex supplement and should be checked for. Many companies leave out the expensive B vitamins, particularly folic acid, biotin and PABA which happen to be amongst the most important.

The Eleven B Vitamins

Vitamin B1 (thiamine)
Vitamin B2 (riboflavin)
Vitamin B3 (niacin)
Vitamin B5 (pantothenic acid or calcium pantothenate)
Vitamin B6 (pyridoxine)
Biotin
Folic acid
PABA
Choline
Inositol
Vitamin B12

Other members of the vitamin B family are not considered as true B vitamins and need to be taken individually. The strengths of the B vitamins contained in a supplement are important and a mega potency vitamin B complex can be considered the most beneficial. Some companies only include three or four B vitamins in a B complex supplement, in minute doses, and fill their tablets out with talc, liquid paraffin, sugar, anti- foaming and anti-caking agents. These should be studiously avoided. It should also be remembered that the B vitamins are largely synergistic, as a family and are more potent when taken together as a complex than when taken in isolation. Exceptions to this rule are pantothenic acid, used in high doses in the treatment of stress conditions

88

and arthritis; nicotinic acid in the treatment of high cholesterol and choline and inositol preferably provided by lecithin, which are used in the reduction of fat and cholesterol levels. Vitamin B6 can be taken in high doses but is preferable in a B complex form as taken alone it can disturb the functions of the other B vitamins, creating some deficiency symptoms. If 100mg B6 is taken daily it may be wise to include a B complex supplement also. The B vitamin taken in a supplement form is more potent when combined with natural food sources of B vitamins such as yeast, wheatgerm and molasses.

OROTIC ACID

Known as vitamin B13 but no longer considered a vitamin. Its chief importance lies in being combined with mineral salts, such as zinc, calcium, magnesium, etc. in order to facilitate their absorption into the system. For this reason some mineral supplements will be described with B13 as a prefix. For example, B13 Chromium indicates that the chromium is blended with orotic acid to increase the minerals rate of absorption into the bloodstream. Orotates are superior to inorganic mineral salts because of their ability to carry mineral salts across cell membranes and their greater rate of absorption through the intestine. Minerals which are combined with orotic acid are expensive but are the best quality available.

VITAMIN B15 (pangamic acid)

A water soluble factor present in the vitamin B complex family. Its main function is the transportation of oxygen from the lungs to the bloodstream and then to the muscles and organs. Vitamin B15 is also useful in detoxifying poisons and free radicals in the system and in stimulating anti-stress hormones. Its use as a carrier of oxygen makes it a popular supplement for athletes. Its other medicinal uses include the treatment of angina, providing higher oxygen levels for the heart muscle and in the treatment of strokes by increasing oxygen uptake to the brain. Pangamic acid is also used in the treatment of exhaustion and fatigue through increasing the transfer of oxygen from the lungs to the bloodstream and organs. Other therapeutic values of vitamin B15 include the treatment of arteriosclerosis, bronchial asthma and diabetes. Best food sources of pangamic acid are: rice, bran, maize, dried brewers yeast, oatflakes, wheatgerm, apricot kernels and wholemeal flour. B15 is also available in supplement form.

BORON

A trace element found principally in fruit, vegetables and nuts principally apples, pears, prunes, tomatoes, raisins, nuts, dates and honey. Boron has been shown to be an essential nutrient frequently lacking in the modern diet. Boron supplementation at low dose levels of 3mg daily reduces the loss of bone minerals, particularly calcium, possibly due to the action of boron in activating vitamin D to increase calcium uptake and due also to its action in stimulating the body's production of sex hormones. Boron is of particular value in the prevention and treatment of osteoporosis in post-menopausal women due to its effect upon bone calcium levels. Professor Bryce-Smith comments 'The findings suggest that supplementation of a low level diet with an amount of boron commonly found in diets high in fruits and vegetables induces changes in post-menopausal women consistent with the prevention of calcium loss and bone demineralisation'. Only low levels of boron are required (approximately 3mgs daily) for prevention of calcium loss and the increased production of sex hormones in post-menopausal women. Boron is also of particular value in the treatment of arthritis. Epidemiological studies indicate that where boron levels are low, incidences of arthritis are high. Doses of 10mg of boron daily have been reported as reducing symptoms in up to 80% of patients. Once symptoms have been relieved the 10mg dose of boron daily can be reduced to 3mg daily. It has been reported that boron supplementation can completely cure arthritis in horses, cattle and dogs.

BIOFLAVONOIDS

Known as vitamin P, bioflavonoids always accompany vitamin C in nature. Richest sources are citrus fruits, apricots, cherries, tomatoes and buckwheat. Bioflavonoids are important in maintaining the health of the blood vessels and capillary arteries, and act as anti-inflammatory factors. They are useful in treating varicose veins, varicose ulcers, haemorrhoids and excessive bruising. The most well-known bioflavonoid is 'rutin', found chiefly in buckwheat and used in the treatment of circulatory disorders due to its action in dilating blood vessels and preventing capillary fragility.

VITAMIN C

Research into man's ancestry, when living in a tropical and sub-tropical environment, has indicated that his intake of vitamin C from plant foods would probably have been between 8 grams and 12 grams daily. Vitamin C is water soluble, is an anti-oxident, promotes iron absorption from the blood, increases the body's resistance to infection, produces anti-stress hormones and helps maintain normal blood cholesterol levels. It also maintains the health of the bones, teeth and sex organs as well as the healthy collagen levels of the body. It reduces the incidence of blood clots in the circulatory system, accelerates healing from surgery and illness, helps heal wounds and burns and is useful in the treatment and prevention of the common cold and other viral infections. It also strengthens the immune system and thereby fortifies the body's front line of defence against allergies, viruses and environmental pollutants. It is also believed that vitamin C has the power to detoxify poisons in the bloodstream, whether due to the action of drugs or environmental pollution, and can remove heavy metals like cadmium and lead from the system. Professor Linus Pauling, a noble prize winner and one of the most eminent scientists of the century, has done much research into vitamin C and is a firm advocate of its use in high therapeutic doses. He maintains that doses of vitamin C (between 2gms and 3gms daily) can act as a preventative of colds and can be used successfully in higher doses in the treatment of colds. He also maintains that vitamin C has a protective action against cancer cells due to its action in strengthening the collagen fibres which holds cells together, making them more resistant to invasive attack from malignant cells. Because collagen is the intercellular cement which holds body cells together and is a natural constituent of healthy skin, vitamin C can preserve the elasticity and youthfulness of the skin and prevent its premature ageing. Professor Linus Pauling advocates taking high doses of vitamin C daily (in doses of 3-4 grams) due, he maintains, to its strongly protective action against cancer. He believes that the adoption of healthy diet and lifestyle and the incorporation of several grams of vitamin C into one's daily diet can help to prevent up to 80% of all cancers. Pauling, himself, takes up to 8 grams of vitamin C daily and is a good advert for his own theories having been born in 1901 and maintaining his health, youthfulness and vitality as he approaches 90 years of age. Vitamin C is also a natural anti-histamine and is therefore useful in the treatment of allergies and hay fever and may be of benefit to schizophrenics as low levels of this vitamin were found in those suffering from this illness. Any form of infection tends to increase the body's needs for vitamin C and higher doses than usual should be taken in order to speed recovery. Deficiencies of vitamin C can cause scurvy, weakness and fatigue, irritability, bleeding gums, pains in the joints and muscles. The best natural sources of vitamin C are fruits and citrus fruits, brussel sprouts and cabbage, rosehip, peppers, tomatoes and most vegetables. However vitamin C is a very unstable nutrient and is easily destroyed in food processing and by oxygen, heat, light and cooking. Some common drugs also destroy vitamin C as also does cigarette smoking, alcohol and the contraceptive pill.

Extra vitamin C is required by those under stress, those with infectious diseases, pregnant women, the elderly and athletes.

Vitamin C supplements should be accompanied by bioflavonoids which always occur with vitamin C in plants and can be taken in powder or tablet form, though preferably without any addition of sugar, preservatives or talc. Vitamin C is extremely non-toxic and can be taken in high doses of several grams daily without any side effects. It is normally available as ascorbic acid or calcium ascorbate which is less acidic and more amenable to higher intakes.

CALCIUM

A mineral salt found in the body in higher quantities than any other mineral. It combines with phosphorus to maintain healthy bones and teeth, controls blood cholesterol levels, assists in the absorption of vitamin B12 and in the process of blood clotting, helps metabolize the body's iron levels, keeps the heart beating regularly and alleviates insomnia. Calcium is often poorly absorbed in women during menopause due to the lowering of oestrogen levels. Extra calcium with vitamin D (which also assists the absorption of calcium) should be taken during this period and ideally continued during the post-menopausal period in order to prevent osteoporosis. Calcium is also used therapeutically during pregnancy and breast feeding in order to maintain adequate levels of this mineral for mother and child and to prevent calcium deficiency disorders in later life. It is also used in the treatment of arthritis, particularly osteoarthritis, and as a detoxifying agent in metal poisoning through lead, cadmium, mercury or aluminium.

A deficiency of calcium can be induced through poor diets, lack of vitamin D, use of the contraceptive pill, and lowered levels of oestrogen at pregnancy (whilst breast feeding and at menopause). Natural sources of calcium are cheese, milk, fish, nuts, beans, root vegetables, eggs, cereal grains and fruits. When the blood levels of calcium fall the parathyroid glands release hormones which activate the release of calcium from the bones and teeth in order to maintain blood levels. If this situation is allowed to continue then clearly dental problems and bone degeneration including osteoporosis and osteoarthritis are likely to occur. Only adequate dietary levels of calcium can prevent this.

The recommended daily intake of calcium is about 1000mg-1200mg of which western diets provide only approximately two thirds of this amount. This discrepancy should be made up either through improved nutrition or through calcium supplementation with added vitamin D. Extra calcium is needed for the following people, those on the contraceptive pill, those taking antibiotics and people using drugs for the treatment of arthritis. Elderly people, those under persistent stress, athletes and consumers of alcohol all have increased needs for calcium.

CALCIUM ASCORBATE

A natural form of vitamin C which can replenish calcium levels which are excreted in the urine due to the chelating action of this vitamin. Calcium ascorbate is less acidic than vitamin C, more easily assimilated and gentler on the stomach.

COD LIVER OIL

This food is a natural source of vitamins A and D and unsaturated fatty acids. It was first used a century ago to cure rickets (being successful due to its vitamin D content). It contains high levels of Omega 3 fatty acids EPA and DHA, which are useful in the prevention and treatment of heart and circulatory disorders due to their ability to thin the blood and prevent its clotting. Experiments were conducted with cod liver oil in the treatment of arthritis and various other complaints and the following results were found. Ninety per cent of osteo and rheumatoid arthritis sufferers showed some benefit within 6 months. There was marked reduction in pain and a diminution in the degree of inflammation and swelling. In other areas there were improvements in complexions, greater alertness and less fatigue, reduction in both cholesterol levels and high blood pressure levels. One tablespoon of cod liver oil was taken daily either alone or in orange juice. It should not be allowed to go rancid and should be consumed rapidly when opened. Keep refrigerated.

CAPRYLIC ACID

This substance is a coconut derivative with anti-fungal properties being used principally in the treatment of candida albicans, a yeast which lives naturally in the intestine but which can spread when the immune system is weakened and unable to keep it in check. Caprylic acid is provided by a supplement named capricin.

CHROMIUM

An essential trace element for both man and animals. Diabetes and heart disease increase when chromium levels in the diet are low. Chromium functions as the glucose tolerance factor (GTF) which stimulates insulin activity. Absorption from food is poor though it occurs in yeast as GTF is 50 times more effective than other forms of chromium. Best food sources are: egg yolk, molasses, brewers yeast, cheese, wholewheat bread. Deficiencies of chromium can be induced through highly refined diets, prolonged slimming diets and alcoholism. Deficiencies of chromium can cause increased cholesterol levels, hardening of the arteries and symptoms of hypoglycaemia including irritability, frustration, intolerance and irrationality, nervous disorders, alcohol intolerance and depression.

COENZYME Q10

This is a nutrient found in every living cell and is essential to life. It is involved in the transfer of oxygen from the bloodstream to the body cells and is essential for the proper functioning of the cells. Low levels of Co Q10 affect the work rate of the cells and can lead to heart disease, mental deterioration and vulnerability to infection. There is some evidence that Co Q10 levels in the body fall as a person ages and that a deficiency of this nutrient may hasten some aspects of the ageing process. Treatment with Co Q10 at levels of 30mg daily divided into 3x10mg doses have been shown to exert a marked anti-ageing influence. Co Q10 occurs naturally in many foods, particularly eggs, soya beans, spinach, brown rice, wheat products and oats. However, it is easily lost in the process of food refining, cooking and storing. In a nutshell Co Q10 fortifies the immune system and protects the body from infection, strengthens the heart and circulatory system, helps to reduce high blood pressure and can be useful in counteracting the effects of ageing. Available in tablet or capsule form normally at strengths of 10mg.

COPPER

This mineral is required to convert iron into haemoglobin, assists the formation of healthy bones and builds up resistance to infection. Natural sources are beans, peas, liver, brewers yeast, nuts, pulses and cereal grains. It also occurs in cigarettes, the contraceptive pill and car exhaust fumes. Deficiencies have occurred in malnourished children, those living on refined diets and in those suffering from prolonged diarrhoea. As a rule, copper deficiency is rare and supplementation is not recommended. Therapeutic uses of copper include the treatment of rheumatoid arthritis.

VITAMIN D

Known as the sunshine vitamin due to the fact that it can only be produced in the body through the action of sunlight on the oils of the skin. For this reason people who have little exposure to sunlight, such as night workers, people who wear excessive clothing and city dwellers (whose intake of the sun's vitamin D producing rays is reduced by smog), should increase their vitamin D dosage. If these skin oils are washed off with soap, the absorption of vitamin D is prevented. When one considers the general lack of sunshine and the need for constant clothing in northern climates it becomes obvious that dietary sources of vitamin D adopt an extreme importance. These are cod liver oil, kippers, mackerel, salmon, sardines, eggs and dairy products. Cod liver oil is the best source of vitamin D with one tablespoon providing 400 i.us the recommended daily dose.

A deficiency of vitamin D causes bow legs and rickets in children and bone pain and brittle bones in adults. Vitamin D also prevents osteoporosis by increasing absorption of calcium. Vitamin D can be toxic in very high doses and 400 i.us-800 i.us daily is all that is required. This can be provided by one or two tablespoons of cod liver oil or 4oz-8oz of oily fish.

DOLOMITE

A naturally occurring supplement of mineral salts, particularly calcium and magnesium. Dolomite is singularly inexpensive and is an excellent source of these two important mineral salts, both being provided in the proper proportions. 3-6 tablets can be taken daily.

VITAMIN E

A fat soluble vitamin which has been credited with miraculous rejuvenating properties. Vitamin E is an anti-oxidant protecting body cells from damage by oxygen, free radicals, and environmental pollutants. It reduces the body's need for oxygen, prevents the blood from clotting, dilates the blood vessels and maintains healthy arteries. For these reasons vitamin E is of particular value in the treatment of heart and circulatory disorders, being used in the treatment of angina and coronary thrombosis. Vitamin E protects polyunsaturated fatty acids in the body, amino acids and vitamin A and increases the virulence of white blood cells in preventing infection. Other therapeutic uses of vitamin E include the treatment of intermittent claudication (pain in the calf muscle caused by poor circulation), strokes, heart attacks, arteriosclerosis, varicose veins, phlebitis and skin ulcers. Vitamin E also has potent healing properties and can be applied directly to scar tissue, burns, stretch marks and sunburn. A lack of vitamin E in the diet can cause lethargy, apathy, decreased interest in sex, loss of concentration and lack of vitality. Vitamin E has also been commonly reported as being able to increase virility and although this is yet unproven, vitamin E is implicated in the health of the glandular system and its production of sex hormones. Vitamin E does appear, however, to be important in maintaining fertility in women and in maintaining normal reproduction. It is credited with the ability to minimise wrinkles and ageing of the skin,, due largely to its role as an anti-oxidant, and can be used both internally and externally for this purpose. Vitamin E has also been found to be particularly beneficial in treating women during the menopause with its symptoms of hot flushes, depression and irritability. Results with vitamin E in the treatment of these complaints have been outstanding. Two Canadian doctors who pioneered research into vitamin E, Dr Evan and Wilfred Shute, successfully treated over 50,000 cases of heart disease with vitamin E in doses ranging from 500 i.us up to 2,400 i.us daily. However, it is not recommended to take such high doses, preferring lower doses of between 200 i.us and 800 i.us daily. It is not recommended to take more than 1,600 i.us daily for long periods, in spite of the relative safety and non-toxic properties of this vitamin. The best food sources of vitamin E are wheatgerm, cold pressed vegetable oils, unprocessed cereal grains, with smaller amounts in green leafy vegetables, nuts, seeds, tomatoes, carrots and eggs. If taking vitamin E as a supplement, always prefer natural vitamin E (denoted by the description d'alpha tocopherol) in preference to synthetic vitamin E (denoted by the term dl'alpha tocopherol), as natural vitamin E is far more active in the body than synthetic vitamin E and is better absorbed and assimilated.

FISH OILS

These have gained importance recently since the discovery of their protective action against heart disease and diseases of the circulatory system. Fish oils are natural sources of essential fatty acids, similar to those found in plant oils (safflower, sunflower) but which also contain 2 fatty acids that are not found in the vegetable kingdom. These are known as the Omega 3 fatty acids which are named EPA and DHA. These fatty acids are known to stimulate the body's production of prostaglandins which effectively thin the blood and inhibit the formation of blood clots in the circulatory system. Tests on Eskimos who obtain high levels of EPA and DHA in their diets showed that healing times in the event of cuts and wounds were markedly slower than healing times in the average westerner. This was because EPA and DHA in the eskimos' diets inhibited the blood clotting mechanism in their circulatory systems. Although they may lose more blood in times of accident and injury, Eskimos are not plagued by heart disease, high fat and cholesterol levels, hardening of the arteries and general circulatory disorders. Cod liver oil and oily fish such as mackerel, salmon and herring are good, natural sources of EPA and DHA. These fatty acids are now available in capsule form (providing 180mg EPA and 120mg DHA per capsule giving a combined intake of 300mg per capsule). Preventative treatment for heart and circulatory disorders requires 3 capsules daily (900mg total EPA and DHA). Those suffering from angina or who have experienced coronary thrombosis or cerebral thrombosis, require 5 capsules daily to prevent further attacks (total EPA and DHA 1500mg).

VITAMIN F

Otherwise known as 'unsaturated fatty acids', including linoleic acid, linolenic and arachidonic acid. Unsaturated fatty acids can reduce cholesterol levels and levels of saturated fat in the system. They thus help to keep the arteries free from cholesterol deposits and maintain the health of the heart and circulation. Unsaturated fatty acids are also important in maintaining the healthy functioning of the glandular system and in correcting skin troubles such as eczema and acne. The best natural sources of essential fatty acids are found in plant foods: wheatgerm, linseed, sunflower seeds, safflower, soya beans, peanuts, walnuts, almonds, avocados or the cold pressed oils extracted from these foods. If sufficient linoleic acid is provided in the diet, the other two fatty acids, linolenic and arachidonic can be synthesised in the system. Oil of evening primrose is one of the best natural sources of vitamin F or essential fatty acids.

GAMMA-LINOLEIC ACID (GLA)

Found in mother's milk and in substantial amounts only in oil of evening primrose seeds, borage oil and blackcurrant and gooseberry seeds. See 'Oil of Evening Primrose'.

FEVERFEW

A plant with a remarkable therapeutic value in the treatment of migraines and arthritis. Known as the aspirin of the 18th century it has been used since the middle ages as a pain relieving herb. Feverfew contains a group of chemicals known as sesquiterpene lactones of which several have been found to be pharmacologically active, the most virulent being parthenolide. Feverfew appears to work like aspirin as an anti-inflammatory agent and by dilating blood vessels. As yet, most of the praise for feverfew has come from testimonial evidence rather than scientific analysis but this makes it no less effective. In 1978 a Welsh doctor's wife Ann Jenkins provoked a storm of publicity by claiming in the national press that she had gained relief from both migraines and arthritis through eating several feverfew leaves daily. Many trials were subsequently carried out and the efficiency of feverfew proven. Results from a clinical trial carried out in the City of London Migraine Clinic showed that benefits occurred in over 70% of sufferers from migraines. Further trials showed that one third of people who maintained the treatment suffered no further attacks. Similar results have occurred in the treatment of osteo-arthritis but, again, evidence is largely of a testimonial character rather than scientific. Many of these testimonials can be found in a book by Dr Stewart Johnson titled simply 'Feverfew', printed by Sheldon Press. One of these testimonial letters is printed here. A retired farmer wrote of his wife and himself:

'Our complaint is arthritis in the fingers, arms and shoulders. A friend of ours was taking feverfew for migraines. She was also crippled with arthritis but after a few months was partly cured of both arthritis and migraines. So we gave it a try for our arthritis which was rather bad with both of us having had it for about 12 years. Since taking feverfew the pain got less until we had no pain. These last 2 years have been without any pain from arthritis. In our opinion it is due to taking feverfew.'

The way that feverfew actually works may yet remain something of a mystery, but there is little doubt that it is an outstanding treatment for migraines if the cause cannot be identified or removed. Feverfew also appears to be successful in treating osteoarthritis, reducing inflammation and easing painful joints though results are not quite as spectacular as in the treatment of migraines. The dose required in the treatment of these 2 complaints is one 200mg feverfew tablet daily which is the equivalent to eating 4 fresh leaves, though these are bitter and acrid to taste. In some persons mouth ulcers can be caused by taking feverfew and these people should stop the medication. Feverfew should not be taken during pregnancy. Feverfew can also be used in the treatment of depression and melancholia, psoriasis and in pain relief, generally due to its ability to inhibit the production of prostaglandins which are involved in the initiation of pain. Again the dose remains at one 200mg tablet daily.

GARLIC

This remarkable herb is an effective antibiotic, antiseptic and general blood cleanser. It contains allicin which has anti-bacterial and anti-inflammatory properties and selenium, which is a natural anti-oxident. It is used in the prevention of colds and infections and to treat asthma and bronchitis. It is also beneficial in reducing high blood pressure due to its action in dilating the blood vessels and improving the general circulation. Garlic is also renowned for strengthening the heart, improving the condition of arthritis and rheumatism due to its anti- inflammatory properties, and in reducing mucous congestion in catarrhal problems. Russian scientists use garlic as an alternative to penicillin, due to its antibiotic action and its ability to cleanse the bloodstream of toxic wastes. For this latter reason garlic is also used in the treatment of acne, boils and pimples and as a general blood purifying agent. Garlic can also neutralise toxic by products which accumulate in the system as a result of the additives, chemicals and preservatives which find their way into the system. It is also believed that garlic can take unwanted metals out of the system, including lead, cadmium and aluminium. It is clearly best to take garlic in its natural form though, due to its offensive odour, most people prefer garlic capsules which dissolve in the intestine rather than the stomach and are virtually odourless. Completely odourless garlic capsules are now also available.

GINSENG

This Chinese root has been used for thousands of years in herbal medicine and is credited with almost mystical powers. It is a stimulant and tonic to the whole system increasing vitality, well being and resistance to infection. It is used by athletes to increase performance and was used by Russian soldiers during the world wars to increase stamina and endurance. Ginseng is used repeatedly in Chinese medicine for its powerful restorative and rejuvenating properties. It is believed to alleviate fatigue and exhaustion and debility in old age and restore sexual energy. The use of ginseng as an aphrodisiac requires some elaboration as it appears to have developed a mystical power in this area of use. Ginseng contains certain compounds which stimulate the body's production of sex hormones and is a general revitaliser of the endocrine system. It contains glycosides which are similar in character to certain body hormones and it appears to be these which possess the tonic and rejuvenating properties of this herb. Ginseng is also useful in times of stress not only for its stimulant properties but due to its action in stimulating the adrenal glands to produce anti-stress hormones. It has also been shown in clinical trials to stimulate the body's production of oestrogen in women, a factor which is of considerable importance during menopause when oestrogen levels tend to fall. Symptoms of the menopause such as hot sweats, irritability and depression were all relieved with ginseng supplementation (at levels of 1200mg Korean ginseng root daily). As a general rule ginseng can be considered as a natural tonic and stimulant. Korean ginseng is the most highly reputed form of ginseng available and comes in root, mixture or tablet form. Siberian ginseng is equally highly rated and much less expensive than Korean ginseng, though it is less explosive and slower acting than its Korean counterpart. It is used principally for its ability to increase stamina and endurance. Available in mixture or tablet form.

GINKGO BILOBA

The world's oldest living tree, dating back 200 million years. Its leaves have considerable medical properties containing pharmacologically active constituents which appear to increase the blood supply to the brain, improve the general circulation, strengthen capillary arteries, and exert a therapeutic influence against the effects of ageing such as forgetfulness, senile dementia, vertigo, tinnitus, poor circulation, loss of hearing and depression. Ginkgo biloba also contains anti-oxidant and anti-inflammatory substances and is useful in improving mental performance.

GLUCOSE TOLERANCE FACTOR (GTF)

This is the active form of chromium with many important functions in the body. GTF helps to control blood sugar and is therefore valuable for diabetics, those prone to hypoglycaemia, and possibly those people with cravings for sugars and sweets. GTF activates insulin to perform its function of removing sugar from the bloodstream. When a deficiency of GTF occurs in the diet more insulin needs to be released by the body to control sugar levels, thus predisposing the individual to maturity onset diabetes. GTF is most active in the body in the form of GTF yeast and may become a necessary supplement for those suffering from diabetes. GTF, in controlling insulin levels and blood sugar levels, may be a supplement of the future in controlling hunger and assisting the body to break down existing body fat. In this way GTF may be a nutrient of immense value in weight control and weight reduction, though scientific analysis has yet to prove this.

IODINE

An essential trace element for man and animals. It is essential in man for its action in maintaining the healthy functioning of the thyroid gland and its hormonal secretions which determines the rate of the body's metabolism.

A lack of iodine causes goitre (swelling around the neck, hence the origin of the expression used to describe inhabitants of an area where iodine is low and goitre is prevalent eg Padiham Thicknecks).

A deficiency of iodine is a worldwide problem, with over 200 million people suffering from diseases related to a lack of this mineral.

Only a tiny amount of iodine is necessary in the bloodstream to maintain the health of the thyroid and its production of the hormone thyroxine. The best natural source of iodine is sea kelp, followed by smaller amounts in fish, vegetables and cereals. A deficiency of iodine can cause an underactive thyroid and a subsequent lack of thyroxine which leads to slow metabolism and overweight conditions, apathy, fatigue and sensitivity to cold. Kelp supplements are inexpensive, are wildely available and can be taken in tablet or powder form.

IRON

This nutrient is essential for life, being involved in the production of haemoglobin (red blood corpuscles) which carry oxygen around the body. Iron helps build resistance to infection, prevents fatigue and impaired growth and mental performance in children. Women lose twice as much iron monthly than men and are prone to dietary deficiencies of this nutrient. A lack of iron in the diet can cause anaemia (which results in tiredness), lack of stamina, headaches, palpitations, insomnia and giddiness. The best natural sources of iron are brewers yeast, wheatgerm, molasses, liver, eggs, nuts, beans, dried fruits and wholegrain cereals. Dietary supplementation with iron is often recommended for women in particular, preferring supplements in the ferrous form eg ferrous gluconate, which is believed to be the best and most readily assimilated form of iron. Ferrous forms of iron do not destroy vitamin E.

VITAMIN K

Functions in the body as an anti-blood clotting agent. This is its sole function. It is frequently given to new born babies due to the poor absorption of this vitamin across the placenta in pregnancy. Best food sources are cauliflower, brussel sprouts, broccoli, spinach, lettuce, cabbage and tomatoes. Vitamin K levels can be reduced by antibiotic therapy and over indulgence in liquid paraffin. Vitamin K is synthesised by intestinal bacteria in the healthy body and supplements are rarely necessary.

KELP

Known otherwise as seaweed. It contains all the minerals, salts and trace elements necessary for health and well-being, but is used principally for its iodine content. Available in powder and tablet form, or as edible seaweed. Kelp is one of the most nutritious foods in existence and is a useful supplement to any diet. All the minerals which occur in sea water are found in healthy human blood providing a possible insight into man's evolutionary origins. The mineral salts of sea water are all contained in abundance in sea-kelp.

EVENING PRIMROSE OIL

For a complete profile on this plant, consult *Evening Primrose Oil* by Judy Graham, published by Thorsons.

The evening primrose plant originated, probably in Central America, some 80,000 years ago and is characterised by its bright yellow flowers. the seeds of the primrose plant are pressed to extract oil and it is this oil - Oil of Evening Primrose - which is known to have great medicinal properties.

Oil of evening primrose, like other plant oils, contains essential fatty acids but is essentially unique in that it contains a substance known as gamma linoleic acid (GLA) which has two indispensible functions. It builds healthy cell membranes and it stimulates the body's production of hormone-like substances known as prostaglandins, in particular prostaglandin E_1, (PGE1). GLA also occurs in moderate amounts in borage, blackcurrant and gooseberry seeds and in higher concentrations in mother's milk. As food sources of GLA are rare it is perhaps not surprising that the body manufactures its own supply of linoleic acid. However the production of GLA in the body is dependant on the function of particular enzymes which convert linoleic acid into GLA. If these enzymes are deficient or operating inefficiently due to poor diet, viral and bacterial infections, stress and overwork, tobacco and alcohol consumption or an excessive intake of sugar and saturated animal fats then the body's conversion of linoleic acid into GLA is hindered resulting in a deficiency. Evening primrose oil, however, is unique in that it already contains gamma linoleic acid in a readily usable form, by-passing the need of the body to produce its own. As mentioned earlier, GLA is produced by the body from linoleic acid, this process often being inhibited by factors such as high cholesterol and fat intakes, excessive alcohol and sugar consumption, stress and the particular hormones that it produces, the effects of ageing, viral infection, radiation and deficiencies of zinc. There is also another factor which blocks the conversion of linoleic acid into gamma linoleic acid which probably affect us all. Natural food sources of vegetable oils such as nuts and seeds (sunflower, safflower, almonds, peanuts, etc) or the cold-pressed vegetable oils from these foods, contain linoleic acid which is readily usable by the body. However, when these oils are processed to remove their smell or increase their shelf life or to converted them into hydrogenated margarine, their linoleic acid content becomes changed to trans linoleic acid, which is recognised as an unnatural substance and does not convert into gamma linoleic acid. Only oil of evening primrose, with its own GLA content, can bypass these problems. Evening primrose oil then, contains essential fatty acids including GLA which, in turn, orchestrates the body's production of prostaglandin PGE1. These substances between them have many important if not miraculous health giving benefits, which are now deserving of further consideration.

PMT and Oil of Evening Primrose

It has been estimated that over 90% of women who suffer from pre-menstrual symptoms such as weight gain, and excessive fluid retention, fatigue, irritability, tender breasts, depression and headaches obtain dramatic relief when administered with oil of evening primrose due to its action in reducing the effects of the female hormone prolactin and other hormones produced by the ovaries.

Two American doctors from a PMS clinic in Massachusettes confirmed the following: "Our clinical research experience has shown that when there is an increase in prostaglandin E1, that is when we are provided the means to produce prostaglandin E1, there is a significant reduction in premenstrual syndrome problems. With a nutritional approach alone, we have a 70% success rate." Dietary recommendations for the treatment of PMT include reducing animal fats, sugar, salt, tobacco, alcohol, tea and coffee and increasing the intake of fruits and vegetables, plant oils from nuts and seeds and the use of whole foods. Evening primrose oil can be taken in doses of between 1-3 grams daily (ie 2-6x500mg capsules daily in divided doses) on the days prior to menstruation, or taken throughout the whole of the menstrual cycle, in doses ranging from 2-4 500mg capsules daily.

Eczema and Oil of Evening Primrose

Deficiencies of essential fatty acids have long been known to produce eczema in both adults and children being characterized by rough scaly skin and a sensitivity to external irritants. Treatment with oil of evening primrose has produced spectacular results though fairly large doses are often frequently required (up to 4 grams daily - 8x500mg capsules). Treatment should be continued for a minimum of 3-4 months before best results can be expected. Children and infants with eczema benefit particularly from primrose oil, though high doses again are required (approximately 3 grams daily). Babies and young children can safely be given primrose oil in the treatment of eczema. If capsules cannot be taken then they can be pricked and the oil incorporated into food or rubbed into healthy skin where it is absorbed into the bloodstream. Remember that mother's milk is the only natural source of high concentrations of GLA other than oil of evening primrose. Breast fed babies are clearly more likely to avoid the onset of

eczema than those reared on cow's milk.
Other complaints such as asthma, hay fever and allergies may be related to eczema in that they usually implicate a faulty immune system as a major causative factor. A deficiency of essential fatty acids in the diet, particularly GLA, may be a contributory factor in this inadequate immune response. GLA stimulates PGE_1 which in turn invigorates the body's production of T. lymphocytes. These have a vital function in the body, maintaining the health and vigour of the immune system and increasing the virulence of scavenging white blood cells in particular.

Rheumatioid Arthiris and Oil of Evening Primrose

Oil of evening primrose appears to be of particular benefit in the treatment of rheumatoid arthritis. GLA invigorates the body's production of prostaglandin PGE1 which has been shown to possess distinct anti-inflammatory properties. In clinical trials about two thirds of patients with mild to moderate symptoms of rheumatoid arthritis experienced dramatic improvements with complete cessation of the progress of their disease when taking primrose oil. Furthermore, most were able to stop taking anti-inflammatory drugs and aspirin, which is welcome due to the action of these medicines in depressing PGE1 levels. Rheumatoid arthritis is considered to be an auto-immune disease where the immune defence mechanism attacks its own joints and connective tissue causing severe inflammation. The reason for this may be that the body is producing too many of the prostaglandins which initiate an inflammatory response, rather than the prostaglandins like PGE1 which have the opposite anti -inflammatory action. Inflammatory prostaglandins are made from arachidonic acid derived from animal foods, particularly meat and dairy products. Anti -inflammatory prostaglandins like PGE1 are derived from essential fatty acids found in the oils from nuts and seeds. It would seem wise in the treatment of rheumatoid arthritis to consume a diet of natural plant foods in preference to a heavy emphasis upon animal foods and to include oil of evening primrose capsules up to 3 grams daily (6x500mg capsules) in divided doses.

Cholesterol and Oil of Evening Primrose

Oil of evening primrose has been found to be particularly effective in reducing high cholesterol levels, in inhibiting the formation of blood clots by reducing the clumping together of blood platelets and lowering blood pressure. It has been reported that oil of evening primrose lowers cholesterol levels as effectively as drugs without any side-effects and with similar success in reducing high blood pressure. Linoleic acid, an essential fatty acid found in plant oils, has long been known to reduce cholesterol levels in man, but its action can be blocked by excessive cholesterol in the diet. GLA, with its stimulation of PGE1 levels, has no such restriction and can reduce cholesterol and blood pressure levels within four weeks and reduce the clotting of platelets in the blood in a matter of hours. Primrose oil should be taken on a daily basis between 2-3 grams daily (4-6 500mg capsules) for a period of several months after which the dose can be reduced.

Alcohol and Oil of Evening Primrose

Primrose oil has been shown to exert a profoundly beneficial action in the treatment of alcoholism and alcohol abuse, particularly in the treatment of liver damage, the alleviation of withdrawal symptoms and the prevention of hangovers. Alcohol in small quantities stimulates the body's production of PGE1 which can induce a sense of mild euphoria. However, alcohol in large quantities, even moderate quantities, has the opposite action and depresses the body's level of prostoglandin E1. Alcohol in small amounts, equivalent to 1 or 2 glasses of beer or wine daily, does appear to have positive health benefits, increasing the life span over non drinkers though the life span is reduced dramatically in heavy drinkers. Alcohol in small quantities does not inhibit any metabolic functions or damage any vital enzymes but in high quantities it prevents linoleic acid being converted into gamma linoleic acid. Consequently a moderate or high consumption of alcohol will induce a significant deficiency of essential fatty acids, and consequently low levels of PGE1, which may account for the severity of the withdrawal symptoms experienced by alcoholics, not to mention the depression experienced in 'boozers gloom'. Low levels of PGE1 have other consequences including a higher risk of heart disease, strokes, high blood pressure and deterioration of the nervous system. Evening primrose oil is of particular benefit to alcoholics and moderate to heavy consumers of alcohol because it elevates the body's levels of PGE1. Oil of evening primrose then can reduce the severity of withdrawal symptoms in alcoholics, it can reduce some of the liver damage and fatty degeneration brought about by alcohol and it corrects a deficiency of essential fatty acids which would otherwise lead to degeneration of the brain and nervous system and premature ageing. It has also been shown to be of particular benefit in preventing hangovers, though evidence for this is of a testimonial nature rather than proven. Doctors researching into the benefits of primrose oil conducted experiments on themselves and found that 4-6 capsules taken before bedtime and after drinking reduced the symptoms of a hangover to a remarkable extent, presumably due to the elevation of PGE1 levels stimulated by gamma linoleic acid.

Hyperactivity and Oil of Evening Primrose

Oil of evening primrose is a useful treatment for hyperactive children and those suffering from excessive thirst, which is a sign of a dietary deficiency of essential fatty acids. Children suffering from hyperactivity frequently suffer from eczema and asthma and often manifest other immune deficiency symptoms such as extreme sensitivity to environmental irritants. This may be due to a lack of the prostaglandin PGE1, a factor which can be corrected with intakes of evening primrose oil at levels of between 2-3 grams daily (4-6 500mg capsules). The hyperactive child should also avoid all preservatives, chemicals and additives in the diet and should be encouraged to adopt a diet of natural foods, with vitamin and mineral supplementation and the inclusion of essential fatty acids in order to build up the response of the immune system.

Benign breast disorders and Oil of Evening Primrose

Primrose oil has also been used successively to treat benign breast disease characterised by tenderness, swelling and breast discomfort. These symptoms appear to be caused by a high intake of saturated fat which blocks the conversion of linoleic acid into gamma linoleic acid, causing menstrual disorders and benign breast problems. Reducing saturated fat in the diet has been shown to reduce the incidences of most cases of benign breast disorders. An interesting consequence of taking oil of evening primrose, though only over long periods of between six months and several years, is an increase in breast size though the reasons for this are yet unknown.

Diabetes and Oil of Evening Primrose

Oil of evening primrose is also beneficial in conditions of diabetes, particularly in alleviating damage to the nervous system (diabetic neuropathy). It is also used in preventing the development of diseases of the eye and circulatory disorders. This slowing down of the progress of diabetic diseases and the general improvement in health experienced by the diabetic due to decreased needs for insulin, appears to result from increased intakes of linoleic acid in the diet or providing oil of evening primrose 2-3 grams daily (4-6 500mg capsules daily in divided doses).

Multiple Sclerosis and Oil of Evening Primrose

In the treatment of multiple sclerosis, geographical studies have shown that MS occurs notably in areas which consume large quantities of animal fat, and rarely occurs in areas where fish and vegetables are prevalent in the diet. This should not be surprising when one considers that the composition of the brain and nervous system is reliant upon an adequate supply of essential fatty acids from dietary sources. Substituting animal fats with vegetable oils from nuts and seeds, adopting a diet of wholesome foods including intakes of oil of evening primrose at levels of 2-3 grams daily (4-6 500mg capsules) should pay dividends in the treatment of multiple sclerosis.

Oil of evening primrose is also used to treat a multiplicity of further conditions, including schizophrenia, where sufferers have been found to have low blood levels of essential fatty acids and PGE$_1$ in their blood, 2-3 grams of primrose oil required daily; certain types of obesity when caused by a metabolic abnormality, best results being with high doses of primrose oil at levels up to 4gs daily (8x500mg capsules) and in treatment of certain forms of cancer as part of a general holistic alternative approach where it appears to have a prohibitive action on the proliferation of the cancer cells. Oil of evening primrose is also valuable in improving the condition and tone of skin, creating a healthy bloom due to its high concentration of essential fatty acids and GLA in particular. Cosmetics made from primrose oil are available and are useful in maintaining the moisture levels and elasticity of the skin. For the treatment of prostate conditions with primrose oil see earlier chapter under 'Prostate Troubles'.

It is clear that oil of evening primrose has turned out to be one of the most outstanding medical discoveries of the century, and its full benefits may not yet be completely understood. Furthermore, due to the fact that primrose oil is a food rather than a medicine, its remarkable benefits are not diminished by any notable side effects. In choosing oil of evening primrose capsules, it is preferable to obtain high quality sources (containing a high fatty acid profile with approximately 10% gamma linoleic acid and 10 i.us of vitamin E) to preserve the quality of the oil. Low quality primrose oil capsules are available, some often blended with poorer quality vegetable oils which do not contain gamma linoleic acid. A reputable herbalist should be able to advise you on this point. It would also seem preferable to use 500mg primrose oil capsules rather than weaker strength capsules as this involves a considerable financial saving in the long term.

Finally a note of caution. Oil of evening primrose is not recommended for epileptics.

LAETRILE

See 'vitamin B17' and the chapter; 'Cancer and Alternative Treatments'.

LECITHIN

The name given to a complex nutrient containing choline, inositol, essential fatty acids and phosphorous. Lecithin was initially discovered in egg yolk as a substance which made possible the mixing of oil and water. Its modern dietary uses are as a fat-fighter or fat emulsifier due to its ability to break down fat and cholesterol levels in the body. Lecithin mobilises fat allowing the body to use it up as energy, it prevents the build up of fat in the body's organs and provides a natural source of polyunsaturated fatty acids.

Lecithin has many therapeutic uses, not surprisingly mostly involved with treatment of blood and circulatory disorders. It is used in the treatment of high blood pressure, to reduce cholesterol and fat levels in the blood, in the treatment of arteriosclerosis and in the prevention and treatment of angina, coronary heart disease, strokes and senile dementia. The best natural sources of lecithin are soya beans, wheat, peanuts, oats, rice, liver, fish and eggs. Lecithin can be taken as a food supplement where it is extracted from the soya bean and is available in granule or capsule form.

MAGNESIUM

An essential mineral salt involved in many bodily processes including the production of energy and the division of cells. Magnesium is also involved in the transmission of nerve impulses, in the body's production of hormones and in the repair and protection of body cells. Magnesium may be lacking from the modern diet due to the use of chemical fertilizers in farming which may prevent the absorption of magnesium by plants. Deficiencies of magnesium can cause fatigue, exhaustion and more particularly are said to cause nervousness and timidity.

Magnesium is nature's own tranquilliser and a deficiency of this may be one of the precipitating factors in the widespread dependency of the population on tranquilisers and sedatives. Deficiencies of magnesium can also cause convulsions, hyperactivity, palpitations and irregular heart beat and muscular tremors. The best natural food sources of magnesium are soya beans, nuts, brewers yeast, brown rice, wholemeal bread, dried fruits and wholewheat flour. Magnesium is useful in the treatment of many common disorders. It has been found to be of particular value in the treatment of pre-menstrual tension, morning sickness, low blood sugar, irregular heartbeats, hardening of the arteries, childhood hyperactivity and insomnia and nervousness. This is due to its calming action on the nervous system.

Of particular interest is the relationship between a low dietary intake of magnesium and high levels of heart disease. Those living in soft water areas have much higher incidences of heart disease due to the lack of magnesium and calcium in the water than those in hard water areas where levels of these mineral salts are higher.

Magnesium forms an important relationship with calcium and supplements of these minerals can be taken together at approximate levels of two parts calcium to one part magnesium. Calcium (500mg) and magnesium (200mg) supplements are available or can be provided by dolomite tablets which are a naturally occurring source of magnesium and calcium in the proper proportions. Dolomite is also inexpensive.

MANGANESE

An essential trace element for man and animals.

Manganese is essential in maintaining a healthy nervous system and bone structure, and in the prodution of energy and female sex organs. Natural food sources are cereals, wholewheat products, nuts, pulses, fruit and green leafy vegetables. Tea drinking provides most of the dietary intake of manganese in the UK (approximately 50%) and deficiencies are rare, unless refined and processed foods form the bulk of the diet.

MOLYBDENUM

An essential trace element for man and animals. Prevents dental caries, maintains male virility and orchestrates the release of iron from storage in the liver.

Natural sources are beans, wheatgerm, liver, soya beans, wholegrain products and buckwheat. Deficiencies are unlikely except in a diet of refined and processed foods and supplements are largely unnecessary.

PHOSPHOROUS

This mineral is a constituent of all plant and animal cells, and due to its wide distribution amongst foods, deficiencies are improbable. Natural sources are brewers yeast, milk, wheatgerm, soya beans, cheese, nuts and cereal grains.

POTASSIUM

A silvery white mineral essential in order for the body to maintain its normal functions. It is widely distributed in food with the best natural sources being fruits, vegetables, dried fruits, soya beans, molasses, nuts, wholegrain cereals, cheese and brown rice. Potassium is often taken out of the body by an excess of sodium (salt) in the diet and also

102

by many medicinal drugs, particularly diuretics. Potassium is an important element, though dietary supplementation is not recommended except in certain circumstances and under professional guidance. The best way to boost potassium levels in the system is to increase fruits and vegetables in the diet and to reduce the intake of salt.

ROYAL JELLY

This is a milky food substance produced by the worker bees for the benefit of their Queen. It is the nutritious properties of royal jelly which account for her greater size and longevity as compared to that of the worker bees from amongst whom she is originally selected.

Royal jelly is a highly nutritious food which contains tiny quantities of most nutrients, including vitamins, minerals, trace elements, enzymes, amino acids and several unidentified ingredients. It is useful as a general tonic and restorative and as a nutritious food supplement but outrageous claims for its medical and therapeutic properties should be ignored.

High quality royal jelly capsules containing wheatgerm oil, in itself a nutritious food, supplying essential fatty acids, are available and can be relatively inexpensive. Avoid expensive forms of royal jelly as these are often extravagantly and unnecessarily over-priced and prefer fresh royal jelly to freeze dried as the freezing process can destroy many of its properties.

The highest quality fresh royal jelly supplements incorporating wheatgerm oil are available, each containing 150mg fresh royal jelly. Stronger capsules are available with up to 500mg fresh royal jelly per capsule.

RUTIN

This is a bioflavonoid known as vitamin P and it is normally found in the presence of vitamin C. Rutin strengthens the walls of the capillary arteries, dilates the blood vessels and is used exclusively in the treatment of circulatory disorders, including poor circulation, high blood pressure and haemorrhoids.

Rutin is also used to treat bleeding gums. Therapeutic doses of this element involve intakes of between 60mg and 600mg and it is preferably taken with vitamin C.

SELENIUM

An essential trace element for man and animals. It functions as an anti-oxident due to its ability to protect body cells from destruction by free radicals and invasive substances which can break down and debilitate these cells. In its role as an anti-oxidant selenium is believed to provide the body with protection from environmental pollution and the corrosive action of oxygen and appears to slow down the process of premature ageing. Selenium is also important in strengthening the immune system and has achieved a degree of importance in the prevention and treatment of cancer. It also helps to detoxify metals like calcium, lead and mercury which find their way into the system through cigarette smoke, smog and environmental pollution. Selenium is irregularly distributed amongst the earth's soils and epidemiological studies have shown conclusively that where soil levels of selenium are low, incidences of both cancer and heart disease are high. Where the soils are high in selenium, incidences of cancer and heart disease are low. In Great Britain, Norfolk has high levels of selenium in the soil and is rewarded with low levels of cancer and heart disease.

Selenium also works as an anti-inflammatory agent and is useful in the treatment of rheumatoid arthritis. It maintains healthy hair, skin and eyesight and is involved in the production of prostaglandins which maintain normal reproductive functions in the male. The best food sources of selenium are organ meats, fish, wholegrain cereals, dairy products, fruits and vegetables. Due to the poor geographical distribution of selenium, however, and to its outstanding importance as an anti-oxident and preventative of cancer and heart disease, food supplements may be necessary. Large quantities of selenium supplementation are not necessary, indeed inadvisable, as this mineral is toxic in high doses. No more than 200mcg should be taken daily with an optimum intake probably being provided by 200mcg in the form of selenium yeast, which increases its absorption and assimilation in the system. Selenium yeast is produced by adding selenium salts to cultivated yeast which then absorbs the trace mineral into its structure. Selenium in yeast is better absorbed and less toxic than inorganic selenium.

TRYPTOPHANE

An amino acid occurring naturally in foods such as milk and cheese and has a pain relieving action. It can lift depression and combat sleeplessness. Some doubt has been cast about the use of tryptophane recently due to its possible contamination during the manufacturing process. A clearer picture should emerge in the future as to the advisability of using tryptophane as a therapeutic agent.

WHEATGERM

The heart of the wheat kernel which contains all the nutrients. Wheatgerm is an outstandingly nutritious food and can be sprinkled readily on most foods, particularly breakfast cereals. Wheatgerm contains high amounts of protein, is high in essential fatty acids, contains choline and inositol (which help breakdown fat and cholesterol levels in the body) and is a rich natural source of vitamin E. Wheatgerm also contains a moderate supply of the B vitamins as well as many mineral salts, trace elements and enzymes including calcium, chromium, iron and manganese. Wheatgerm is one of the most nutritious foods available, is extremely versatile and can be incorporated easily into any diet. It is also extremely inexpensive.

YEAST

Dried brewers yeast is quite conceivably the most nutritious food available to man. It is a plant food containing 40% protein and an abundance of vitamins, minerals, enzymes and trace elements. It is particularly rich in members of the B vitamin family and is a natural tonic for the nervous system and for those suffering from nervous debility and fatigue. Brewers yeast is also particularly rich in chromium and selenium and contains high quantities of choline and inositol, iron and calcium. Brewers yeast is a welcome and extremely nutritious addition to any diet and like wheatgerm is particularly inexpensive. It is probably best taken added to fruit and vegetable juices in doses of one tablespoon daily, though more can readily be taken. Available in powder or tablet form. One tablespoon of brewers yeast powder is equal to approximately sixty tablets and is the preferred form of use.

ZINC

An essential trace element for man and animals. Zinc is often lost in the refining and processing of food, the manufacture of white flour from wholewheat flour causes a 77% loss of zinc while the processing of brown rice into white rice causes an 83% loss of zinc. Zinc is important for protein synthesis, the manufacture of insulin, the development of the brain and nervous system, the health of the prostate gland, the healthy functioning of the liver and the physical, mental and sexual development of adolescents. A lack of zinc can cause retarded growth and inhibit the development of the sexual and reproductive organs. A deficiency can cause eczema, post natal depression, congenital abnormalities in the new born and loss of taste and smell. Zinc can also help reduce cholesterol deposits, promote mental alertness, speed up the healing of wounds and injuries, and can be used in the treatment of psoriasis, acne rosacea, schizophrenia and hyperactivity in children. Zinc can be used in the treatment of anorexia nervosa by restoring to normal the individual's sense of taste and smell, the loss of which appears to be an important factor in the progression of the disease. Zinc has also been shown to be of considerable benefit in treating the common cold if taken in the form of zinc gluconate lozenge, in strengths of 25mg per tablet. The lozenge must be sucked to be of benefit, releasing the zinc to enter the mucous membranes where it acts as a natural antibiotic capable of inhibiting the replication of common cold viruses and arresting the duration of the common cold. For purposes other than the treatment of the common cold zinc is best taken in the form of zinc gluconate or zinc orotate tablets in doses ranging from 25mg to 100mg. Zinc orotate supplements where the zinc is combined with orotic acid are believed to be the best absorbed and are usually available in 100mg strength, one tablet daily is all that is required. It is not required that zinc supplements should be taken indefinitely as only certain levels of zinc are required in the body. Intakes superfluous to requirements are unnecessary and zinc supplementation can be reduced after several months. Alternatively zinc supplements can be taken once or twice weekly.

The need for supplements to a modern diet

The justification for the taking of vitamin and mineral supplements comes from the imperfections of both our environment and our lifestyles. Plant foods are grown on devitalised soils with artificial fertilisers and frequent administrations of pesticides and toxic chemicals. Animals destined for the slaughter house are fattened with injections of growth hormones and natural wholesome foods are often heavily processed and refined removing their important nutrients. Cooking further destroys the nutritional value of foods, whilst the use of tobacco, alcohol and many medicinal drugs often further deplete the body's supplies of vitamins and minerals. As a general rule supplementation of the diet with minerals is required only to correct a dietary deficiency of these elements. Once the deficiency has been corrected there is little justification in taking higher doses of minerals than are needed to maintain the body's requirements. Minerals are not used in high doses for therapeutic treatments of diseases. Vitamin supplementation is, however, used both to correct bodily deficiencies of vitamins and to treat various complaints and illnesses in high therapeutic doses. For example, high doses of vitamin E are used in the treatment of heart and circulatory disorders. As a general rule, due to the poor quality of modern food and the deleterious actions of environmental pollution, stress, alcohol and tobacco consumption on nutrient levels in the body it may be wise to include a high quality vitamin and mineral supplement in the diet as a form of insurance against any possible dietary deficiency.

It should also be mentioned that vitamins and minerals are largely synergistic. Many vitamins and minerals are also interdependent and cannot function without the presence of their dependant factor. This is a further good reason for preferring a high quality vitamin and mineral combination rather than attempting the impossible task of taking all necessary nutrients individually. The best vitamin and mineral supplements available in Great Britain are manufactured by Larkhall Laboratories and presented as 'Cantamega 2000'. This is the strongest and most comprehensive vitamin and mineral supplement on the market, containing all nutrients in high doses, including a potent combination of all eleven members of the B vitamin family. 'Cantamega 1000' is a less potent vitamin and mineral supplement but contains all nutrients in moderate doses. Investigation and research into the quality and credibility of vitamin and mineral supplements in the UK repeatedly finds that Cantamega 2000 and 1000 vitamin and mineral supplements are the best quality and value for money. They are also cut into divided doses for children. Once a high grade vitamin/mineral supplement has been established it is then possible to make whatever further nutritional additions are considered necessary. Vitamin A (beta carotene) is useful for its protective action against certain forms of cancer and can be provided by either carrot juice or vitamin supplementation. The B complex family is destroyed by cooking, alcohol, stress, antibiotics, sugar and are heavily refined from foods. It can be provided in small quantities by the inclusion of both wheatgerm and brewers yeast in the diet or in higher potencies in a B complex formula, or in the multi vitamins and minerals in Cantamega 2000.

Vitamin C is an outstandingly valuable nutrient and is highly recommended as a nutritional supplement due to its poor distribution amongst modern foods and its easy destruction in cooking and storage. Vitamin C is a natural anti-oxidant, reducing the damage to cells from oxygen and free radicals. It maintains collagen levels in the body preserving the elasticity of the skin. It also promotes resistance to disease and has a preventative value in cancer. Vitamin C supplements are relatively inexpensive and should be taken if possible without sugar, talc, filling or binding agents. Take preferably with bioflavonoids as these substances occur with vitamin C in nature. Vitamin D is essential for the absorption of calcium and can be provided by sunshine and cod liver oil. Vitamin E is an anti-oxidant which preserves the youthfulness of body cells, prevents the blood from clotting and has a general therapeutic action in the prevention and treatment of circulatory disorders. It is available in capsule form preferring the natural form of vitamin E (d'alpha tocopherol) to the synthetic.

Essential fatty acids can be provided by including nuts, seeds and their cold-pressed oils in the diet or by the use of oil of evening primrose capsules. Mineral salts require some consideration due to their extreme importance in the prevention of certain diseases. Kelp provides a wide range of mineral salts in low doses and is a useful general supplement. Calcium may require supplementation in tablet form, containing vitamin D to facilitate absorption, particularly amongst women during the menopause when low levels of oestrogen inhibit the absorption of this mineral. Calcium throughout the menopause or prior to its onset is a protective against the development of osteoporosis (crumbling of the bone). Iron supplementation may be necessary again particularly amongst women whose losses of this mineral are much greater than in men. Iron can be provided by ferrous gluconate supplements preferably although the use of iron rich foods like blackstrap molasses, liver and yeast may be sufficient.

Selenium is an extremely important mineral due to its poor geographical distribution in the earth's soils, so may be lacking in some diets. It is important as a protective agent against cancer and heart disease. It would appear to be wise to include a selenium supplement in the diet preferably in the form of selenium yeast at levels of 200mcg daily. This is a low dose but all that is required. Calcium and magnesium work together in the system and are particularly important in preventing heart disease. Soft water areas of the country which contain low levels of magnesium and calcium have much higher incidences of heart disease than hard water areas which supply these minerals. This relationship between low levels of calcium and magnesium and heart disease has been proven conclusively and the information has been available for more than 15 years. It is pertinent to ask why the medical authorities in this country have shown such little interest in this relationship and the dissemination of this information to the public preferring the use of surgery and medicine once heart disease has been established. Calcium and magnesium supplements are available and should be taken in doses of two parts calcium and one part magnesium e.g. calcium 500mg and magnesium 200mg. These are inexpensive and require only one or two tablets every few days. Dolomite is also a good natural source of calcium and magnesium in the right proportion and is extremely inexpensive.

Zinc may be undersupplied in the modern diet due to the refining and processing of food and a supplement may be advisable for certain periods rather than indefinitely. Zinc orotate supplements are the best although zinc gluconate is well absorbed and extremely inexpensive. Most other mineral salts will be adequately supplied particularly by a diet of natural foods especially if including wheatgerm and brewers yeast as a regular feature. Multi-minerals in orotate form are available though expensive. Natural and inexpensive forms of mineral supplementation include the use of kelp, dolomite and blackstrap molasses.

It should go without saying that vitamins and mineral supplementation is of strictly secondary importance to the adoption of a natural diet of plant foods, including fruit, vegetables, nuts, seeds, beans, cereal grains of wheat, oats, barley, brown rice and the inclusion of low fat dairy products and nutritious foods such as wheatgerm, kelp, brewers yeast and molasses.

CHAPTER NINE

Herbs and their uses

Herbs, roots and barks have been used for thousands of years to provide medicines for the benefit of humanity, and at present their use appears to be undergoing a resurgence in popularity. Below is a simple list of common herbal remedies, though it is always wise to consult a registered medical practitioner before embarking on self-treatment for serious ailments. Herbal medicines are normally prepared by putting 1 oz of herb to 1 pint of boiling water and allowing to infuse for 5-10 minutes. The liquid can then be drunk (3-4 wineglassfulls daily). Roots and barks require simmering for 10 minutes in order that their healing properties be extracted.

This glossary of herbs is necessarily short, as there are approximately a quarter of a million identified herbs and many more not yet identified.

Agrimony

Used as a tonic and a diuretic, for sickness, diarrhoea and headaches.

Angelica

Relieves flatulence, stimulates the vital powers, activates the circulation and regulates menstruation.

Aniseed

Used as an expectorant in cough mixtures to break up phlegm, to counteract flatulence and in the treatment of bronchitis and asthma.

Asafetida

A gum resin used as a stimulant, an expectorant in cough mixtures and as a treatment for infantile convulsions and flatulence.

Barberry Bark

Used to treat jaundice, liver complaints, biliousness and general dibility.

Bayberry Bark

A powerful stimulant and tonic. When combined with cayenne, it induces perspiration and is used in the treatment of chills and clamminess.

Belladonna

Known as Deadly Nightshade. Used to relieve pain and is a sedative. Used as a treatment for coughs and whooping cough.

Benzoin

A gum used as an expectorant in coughs and bronchitis.

Bladderwrack

Used in the treatment of obesity as an anti fat agent and a diuretic.

Blood Root

A stimulant and tonic and expectorant of great value in chest diseases, pneumonia and bleeding of the lungs.

Boldo Leaves

A tonic, stimulant and diurhetic

Boneset

Chiefly used in cases of fever, colds and catarrh.

Borage

A natural diuretic. Promotes perspiration and is used in coughs, colds, bronchitis and in the treatment of skin disease.

Broom

Diuretic and purgative.

Buchu

Diuretic, induces perspiration. Stimulant, with a direct action on the urinary organs. Used to treat inflammation of the bladder.

Burdock

Diuretic and blood purifier. Used freely in the treatment of boils, eczema, psoriasis and rheumatism.

Cajuput

The oil is used as a stimulant and for relief of pain, internal and external. Taken a few drops on sugar, it is used to treat flatulence and colic.

Calamus Root

Used as a treatment in flatulence and dyspepsia.

Caraway

A seed used as a stimulent and used to expel flatulence.

Catmint

Induces perspiration and is used in the treatment of colds and fevers. Also useful in treating hysteria and restlessness.

Cayenne

A powerful stimulant and tonic. It produces a natural warmth and improves the circulation. Used in the treatment of colds.

Celandine

A blood purifier, diuretic and purgative. The fresh juice of the plant removes corns and warts.

Celery Seeds

Used to expel flatulence and in the treatment of rheumatism.

Centaury

Used in conjunction with Barberry Bark in cases of jaundice. Used extensively in dyspepsia and weak digestion.

Chamomile Flowers

A tonic and natural sedative used to induce sleep and to combat hysteria and nervousness. Can be applied externally for toothache, earache and neuralgia. A natural aid to digestion.

Chickweed

Generally used in ointments for carbuncles, abscesses and skin eruptions.

Clivers

Diuretic and tonic. Used in obstructions of the urinary organs.

Black Cohosh

An emmenagogue, inducing the menstral flow. Used in the treatment of whooping cough.

Coltsfoot

An expectorant used in cough medicines.

Comfrey

Contains a substance called allantoin, a noted healing ingredient. Used in the treatment of chest complaints and as a healing agent in the treatment of stomach ulcers and inflammation. Used externally to promote the healing of wounds and sprains.

Cranesbill

Used to treat diarrhoea and to stop internal or external bleeding. A natural kidney tonic.

Damiana

Used as an aphrodisiac and tonic, and for its beneficial action on the reproductive organs.

Dandelion

A diuretic and tonic and is used chiefly in the treatment of liver and kidney disorders and as a blood purifier.

Echinacea

Used to treat inpurities of the blood. A potent blood cleanser in boils and carbuncles.

Elder Flowers

Induce perspiratiron and are used in the

treatment of colds, fevers and influenza.

Elecampagne Root

Induces perspiration and is a natural expectorant. Used in the treatment of chest and bronchial complaints.

Eye-bright

Used as a remedy in weakness of the eyes. It is frequently combined with Golden Seal and made into an infusion for bathing the eyes.

Fennel

Used to combat flatulence and stomach disorders.

Fenugreek Seeds

Useful as a poultice in abscesses and boils and on inflamed conditions of the stomach.

Gentian Root

A tonic. Used in all cases of weakness of the digestive system and general dibility.

Ginger

A stimulant and expectorant used in the treatment of colds.

Ginseng

Tonic and stimulant.

Golden Rod

A diuretic. Used in conditions of ulceration of the bladder and intestines.

Golden Seal Root

Used to treat inflammatory conditions of the digestive system, particularly ulcers and digestive dibility. Used externally as a treatment for eye infections.

Gravel Root

Used as a diuretic and in the treatment of stones in the bladder, as well as kidney troubles.

Guarana

A tonic and stimulant due to the caffeine content of the seeds. Enjoying modern day popularity.

Hawthorn

Used in the treatment of high blood pressure and is a cardiac tonic.

Hemlock

Sedative and a pain killer.

Horehound

An expectorant used in most herbal cough mixtures.

Hyssop

A stimulant and a good remedy for coughs, colds and lung complaints.

Iceland Moss

Used to improve appetite and to treat catarrh and chronic bronchitis.

Ipecacuahna

Used in most modern cough mixtures as an expectorant, and in cases of colds and dysentry.

Kola Nut

A nerve stimulant, aphrodisiac and cardiac tonic. Contains caffeine. An excellent remedy for diarrhoea.

Ladies Mantle

Used as a cure for excessive menstruation.

Lime Flowers

Tonic, stimulant and strengthens the nervous system. Used also in restlessness, hysteria and catarrh.

Linseed

Used largely in cough mixtures and in the treatment of chest complaints.

Liquorice

Root - a well known expectorant used widely in cough and bronchial medicines.

Lobelia

Causes vomiting (emesis) and is used in bronchial complaints. It removes mucous rapidly from the system and is especially valuable in the treatment of whooping cough and asthma.

Mandrake

A purgative and glandular stimulant.

Marigold

Induces perspiration and is a stimulant. Used as a healing agent in local applications.

Marshmallow

Used in the treatment of coughs and bronchitis. Also useful as a healing agent in the treatment of ulcers and as a poultice to remove the most obstinate ulcers.

Meadowsweet

Used to treat diarrhoea in children. A diuretic.

Motherwort

A tonic and nervine used also in cases of cardiac debility. It promotes the menstrual flow and allays nervous irritability.

Muira Puama

Aphrodisiac and nerve stimulant.

Myrrh

A gum resin which acts as a stimulant and tonic and is a healing agent in inflammatory conditions of sore throat and ulcers.

Nettle

A tonic and diuretic.

Nutmeg

Expels flatulence and is used in the treatment of nausea and vomiting.

Oat Seeds (Avena Sativa)

A nerve tonic and stimulant. A restorative in all cases of nerve exhaustion and debility.

Paraguayan Mate Tea

A stimulant and diuretic. Contains caffeine.

Parsley Piert

Used in all cases of bladder and kidney complaints.

Pellitory of the Wall

A laxative and diuretic used in the treatment of stones and gravel normally in conjunction with parsley piert.

Pennyroyal

An emmenagogue used to induce the menstrual flow.

Peppermint

Used in the treatment of nausea, flatulence, sickness and vomiting, and in cases of indigestion and hyperactivity.

Periwinkle

Used in the modern day treatment of diabetes.

Pilewort

Used in the treatment of piles. Take as an infusion. Externally it can be used as an ointment.

Pleurisy Root

Promotes perspiration and is used in the treatment of pleurisy where it relieves difficulty of breathing. Used in all chest ailments and is a natural expectorant.

Poke Root

Used to treat dyspepsia and chronic rheumatism.

Pulsatilla

Used to treat nervous exhaustion and is an antispasmodic to relieve cramps and pains.

Quassia

Used in the treatment of dyspepsia and digestive debility. Useful also in the treatment of worms.

Queen's Delight

A blood purifier and tonic used principally to remedy impure conditions of the blood.

Raspberry Leaves

A useful gargle for sore mouths and throats. Used by pregnant females to give strength and for easy parturition.

Red Clover

A sedative and alterative. A remedy for bronchial coughs and whooping cough.

Red Sage

An excellent gargle for sore throats and tonsils.

Rosmary

Promotes perspiration and is a natural tonic. Excellent in the treatment of stomach troubles and as a nerve tonic. used externally as an infusion for healthy hair.

Sarsparilla Root

A blood purifier and general restorer of the system. Used in the treatment of skin disorders and rheumatism.

Sassafras

A stimulant, promotes perspiration, and is a diuretic. Used in the treatment of skin eruptions, gout and rhematism.

Saw Palmetto

A natural tonic and aphrodisiac. The berries are used in the treatment of all wasting diseases as well as having a profound effect on glandular secretions. They are renowned for their strength giving properties.

Scullcap

A tonic to the nervous system and an antispasmodic. Possible the finest nerve tonic available. used in the treatment of hysteria, convulsions and nervous debility.

Senna

A laxative and cathartic.

Shepherds Purse

Chiefly used in the treatment of kidney complaints.

Skunk Cabbage

An expectorant used in cough mixtures and as a remedy for asthma and bronchitis.

Slippery Elm

A most valuable soothing and healing agent which reduces inflammation and is also a highly nutritious food. Can be used in all cases of stomach inflammation and bleeding and general debility.

Southernwood

Induces the menstrual flow. Used also to treat worms in children.

St Johns Wort

Used in the treatment of lung and chest disease. Used externally as a healing application for wounds and sores.

Tansy

A tonic and emmanagogue. Expels worms in children.

Thuja

Used as an external application for warts and fungal growth.

Tolu Balsam

Stimulant, tonic and expectorant used in coughs and bronchial mixtures.

Tormentil Root

Used in cases of relaxed bowels and diarrhoea.

Uva Ursi

Used in the treatment of kidney troubles and disorders of the urinary system.

Valerian Root

Pain-relieving, antispasmodic and nerve tonic. Used in all cases of nervous debility and to promote sleep.

Vervain

Induces perspiration, a nerve tonic and causes vomiting. Used in the treatment of fevers and colds.

Violet Leaves

Used historically to alleviate pain and frequently to arrest the progress of cancerous growths. Used also as an expectorant.

Wild Carrot

A diuretic and stimulant, used in the treatment of water retention, bladder and kidney troubles.

Willow Bark

Aspirin was first discovered in this bark which is used for pain relief and in the treatment of rheumatism and diarrhoea.

Witch Hazel

An astringent skin tonic, particularly useful in checking haemorrhages and in the treatment of piles.

Yarrow

A stimulant and tonic and diaphoretic (induces perspiration). Useful in the treatment of colds and fevers, it opens the pores and pirifies the blood.

Yellow Dock

Very rich in iron, a laxative, tonic and blood purifier. Used freely in rheumatism and skin diseases, piles and biliousness. Useful in the treatment of ezcema.

CHAPTER TEN

A brief guide to Aromatherapy

When flowers, herbs, roots and barks are subjected to a process of distillation, their volatile oils are captured and known as Essential Oils. These are then used in Aromatherapy to influence both physical and emotional states and to invigorate the body's own healing force. Aromatherapy oils can be used in a variety of ways; a few drops on a handkerchief or tissue can be used for inhaling, or they can be added to vegetable oils and used for massage, or they can be put in the bath to create a subtle mood changing aroma, or they can simply be used as perfume. It must be remembered that aromatherapy oils are particularly concentrated and should rarely be taken internally.

Below is a list of the most common oils used in aromatherapy and their therapeutic uses.

Basil

Used as a stimulant for the nervous system and to counteract mental fatigue, loss of concentration and general exhaustion. Add several drops to a tissue and inhale. Can be used with a carrier oil as a massage.

Bergamot

Used to flavour Earl Grey Tea and to treat depression and anxiety. A relaxant and mild antiseptic. Used also as an inhalation for its benefits in the treatment of indigestion and flatulence.

Black Pepper

A hot stimulating oil which causes dilation of local blood vessels and is therefore useful as a massage in the treatment of muscular aches and pains. It also stimulates the mind and circulation and improves the digestion.

Cajuput Oil

Used in the treatment of colds, coughs and respiratory difficulties, normally in inhalations. A few drops on the bath promotes perspiration.

Cedarwood

An antiseptic and sedative.

Chamomile

A natural anti-inflammatory with an analgesic action. Can be used as an inhalant to relax the system, and as a treatment for diarrhoea, teething pains and earache. Chamomile oil is a sedative and anti-depressant and induces sleep.

Camphor

A stimulant used in the treatment of coughs and colds, usually as an inhalant. Frequently used with a carrier oil as a chest rub. Not to be used by epileptics.

Cinnamon

Used as a treatment in digestive ailments and for its aromatic scent.

Clary Sage

A natural sedative and anti-depressant used to treat period pains and irregular periods. Used as an inhalation to treat nervousness and help hysteria.

Clove

Used for treatment of toothache and is a powerful antiseptic.

Coriander

A refreshing stimulant.

Cypress

A few drops in the bath help relaxation. Used to treat coughs and as an astringent.

Eucalyptus

Used in inhalations in the treatment of colds, flu, catarrh and sinusitis, fever and congestive headaches. Can be used when diluted with oil as a rub for rheumatism and chest complaints.

Fennel

A diuretic used also in the treatment of digestive trouble. Should not be used in pregnancy or on young children.

Frankincense

Used as an inhalant for all catarrhal conditions, coughs and shortness of breath. Used in anti-wrinkle prepartions for its action in preserving the youthfulness of skin. It is also an aid to meditation.

Geranium

A sedative used in the treatment of anxiety states. Useful also when applied externally in the treatment of wounds.

Ginger

A powerful oil to be used sparingly. Useful in the treatment of rheumatism and arthritis. One or two drops only can be used in the bath.

Hyssop

Used to stimulate the mind and nervous system inducing clarity and alertness. Can be inhaled for bronchial troubles, and to counteract flatulence. Not to be used by epilectics.

Jasmin

A very expensive oil reputed to possess aphrodisiac properties. Useful as an anti-depressant. Can be used as a massage oil.

Juniper

The oil extracted from juniper berries is a natural kidney tonic and diuretic and is used to make gin to which it imparts it's characteristic scent. Can be used as a massage oil for skin disorders incuding eczema and dermatitis.

Lavender

Can be used as an inhalant for its sedative and toning action and in the treatment of depression, insomnia and exhaustion. A few drops in the bath will induce relaxation and sleep. Used in massage oils, it is beneficial in the treatment of muscular and rheumatic pains.

Lemon

Used as an astringent to treat oily skin, and to help remove warts and verrucas.

Lemongrass

Used principally for its aromatic fragrance.

Marjoram

An inhalant for colds, headaches and insomnia. Used in massage oils for treatment of rheumatism and sprains. Valuable in the treatment of anxiety.

Marigold

A healing oil which reduces inflammation.

Melissa

Used for its fragrant scent and in the treatment of allergies and as a general tonic.

Myrrh

Can be used in diluted form to treat haemorrhoids, mouth ulcers, wounds and sores. Greek soldiers always took myrrh into battle to treat wounds. Can be used internally to stimulate the appetite and combat flatulence.

Neroli (Orange Blossom)

Used for its aromatic fragrance and its power to induce relaxation. Useful in the treatment of stress and depression.

Orange

Imparts vitality and good spirits.

Patchouli

An ahrodisiac widely used in perfume and aftershave. A rich earthy sent useful for healing chapped skin. A natural sedative and antiseptic.

Peppermint

Used as an inhalant for fever, colds, influenza, indigestion, diarrhoea and nausea. Most commonly used to treat digestive upsets, and is invigorating when used in the bark. Improves the circulation and is a natural tonic.

Pine

Use as an inhalation for colds and coughs, removes aches and pains when put in the bath.

Rose Otto

An anti-depressant used also in perfumes.

Rosemary

A stimulant to the nervous system improving vitality, concentration and memory. Used in hair tonics. Useful as an inhalation for bronchial troubles.

Rosewood

Used principally for its refreshing scent.

Sandalwood

Used to treat digestive troubles and is a natural astringent and antiseptic in the treatment of skin complaints. Widely used in perfumes, and as a gargle for through infections.

Thyme

Used in the treatment of asthma, influenza and flatulence. Can be used externally as a massage for rheumatism and muscular pains. Useful in the treatment of sore throats and bad breath.

Ti-Tree

A powerful antiseptic and anti viral agent. At the outset of flu or cold symptoms, put 3-4 drops of oil in the bath.

Ylang Ylang

An aphrodisiac widely used in perfumes. A natural sedative, relaxant and anti-depressant. Highly recommended in calming the nervous system in stress situations. Can be dabbed on the wrist or behind the ear.

Parsley
(Petroselinum Crispum)

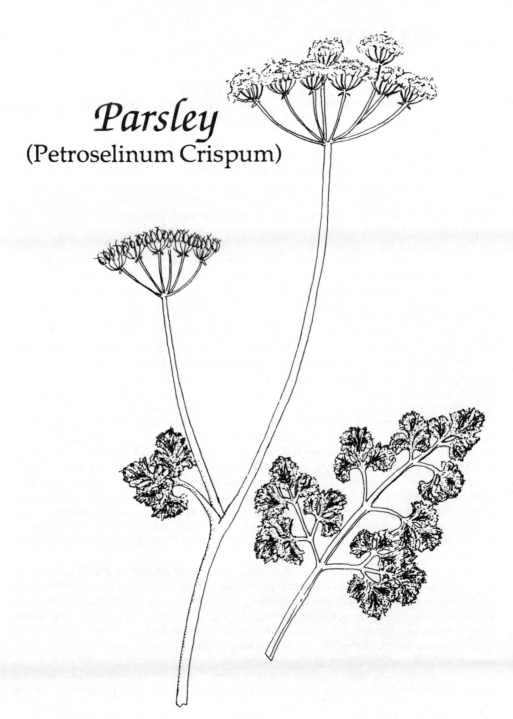

CHAPTER ELEVEN

The Politics of Health

It should be clear from earlier chapters that whereas orthodox medicine tends to view disease as a localised entity and the body as a collection of parts, the philosophy of natural medicine views disease as a breakdown of the constitution as a whole and as such attempts to treat the whole person, body, mind and soul when illness occurs. In the treatment of disease natural medicine recognises the importance of re-habilitating the whole system through observance of the eight healing forces of nature and of liberating the body's own healing power, an innate life-force of the system which operates as a self-rejuvenating and self-healing energy. By removing the causes of disease, natural medicine allows the body the opportunity to work towards a condition of health and harmony. This is the central and intractable core of alternative medicine. Health can only be maintained or re-built through respect for the elements of nature and her healing forces of food, air, water, sunshine, sleep and rest, exercise and positive thought/emotional poise. Orthodox medicine over the last 50 years has largely ignored these principles, preferring to dispense vast quantities of pharmaceutical drugs and medicines in the treatment of disease, without making any concessions towards the philosophy of nature-cure or towards the all important role of preventative medicine and health education. It is suggested by nature cure practitioners, including Harry Benjamin who wrote the renowned encyclopedia on natural medicine entitled *Everybody's Guide to Nature-Cure*, that the sum total contribution of orthodox medicine in the treatment of disease is to worsen the condition of humanity rather than to improve it. The inclination of the medical profession towards dosing the population with drugs and mixtures rather than removing the causes of disease reveals further that orthodox medicine has compromised its principles and bent its moral duty to the wholesale promotion of pharmaceutical medicines in the treatment of disease to the neglect of the principles of natural healing and health education and in doing so have undermined their own credibility and given rise to doubts about the sincerity of their motives.

There are some valuable and admirable aspects to orthodox medicine but its approach to the treatment of disease is generally not one of them. There is little doubt that we live in an imperfect world, abusing the laws of nature with little inclination towards change, thereby frequently rendering medical intervention necessary. Where modern science is successful, whether it be in the treatment of accidents and emergencies, heart, lung or kidney transplants, hip and joint replacements, maternity care, orthopaedics, general surgery or the treatment of infectious diseases, etc, or in whatever form or manner modern medicine benefits the human condition or improves the quality of an individual's life, then the medical profession and its practitioners deserve our uninhibited admiration and gratitude. It is only possible to be thankful and deeply indebted towards medical staff where their skill and dedication are extended to improving the human condition, health and preserving the gift of life. However, since the beginnings of the Health Service in post war years, modern medicine has devoted itself to the wholesale dispensing of drugs and medicines to treat all ailments. There is no concession to the value of natural medicine or the environmental causes of disease and the power of the body to heal itself. The importance of diet and lifestyle in the prevention and treatment of disease throughout has been completely dismissed, with lip-service alone being paid to the value of health education and preventative medicine. It was shown conclusively in the 1920s from experiments with the Hunza diet, mentioned at the beginning of this book, that diet and lifestyle were the single most important factors in the prevention and treatment of disease. The Hunza's showed that by living in harmony with the laws of nature, complete health and vitality, free from disease was possible. This type of information and the impetus it should have provided for further scientific investigation has been completely ignored in favour of pharmaceutical treatments for conditions of ill-health. If the cause of disease is not removed from the individual's lifestyle, whether it be dietary or environmental in origin, then disease will stay with us, along with the toxic side-effects from prescribed medicines. Doctors themselves are principally not to blame for this state of affairs as their capability is limited by the prejudiced slant of their medical training which emphasises pharmaceutical solutions in preferance to a deeper understanding of the dietary and environmental causes of disease. Many are further abused by the system in the colossal degree of stress and overwork imposed upon them with the inevitable toll of stress related illnesses which ensue.

Health can be built and maintained only through harmony with the elements and observance of natural laws and not through the ingestion of largely poisonous drugs and mixtures. Drug companies might wish to be seen as pioneers of research, conferring great benefits on humanity, but the truth is something different. It is the endless search for profit which motivates them and while many drugs are useful it must be understood that the patient's welfare is of secondary concern.

For example, drugs which have been shown to possess debilitating side effects that are banned in Europe and America are frequently shipped to Third World countries where they are indiscriminately used. In Asia the lack of education of the population is cruelly exploited by drug companies and multi-national businesses alike. Mothers are encouraged through high powered marketing and advertising to feed their babies on powdered milk in preference to breast milk, with the consequence that in mixing the powdered milk with contaminated water their babies often develop illnesses, among them a debilitating form of diarrhoea from which they frequently do not recover. The drug companies' response is to promote a drug called 'indocid' for the treatment of diarrhoea, and this in itself can cause intestinal paralysis and a painful, protracted death.

In the treatment of infectious diseases throughout history improved sanitation and hygiene have triumphed over the use of medicine. Modern antibiotics are not the blessing they are frequently exhorted to be, having the action of destroying healthy cells and weakening the immune system, rendering the individual more prone to re-infection and providing the impetus for other diseases. The short term value of most synthetic medicines is largely confined to their action as palliatives and pain relievers rather than cures, with their long term action invariably weakening the health of the individual. The Natural Medicines Society, a body dedicated to the propagation of health education and the protection of herbal and natural medicines from attack by government legislation has presented the following facts about the pharmaceutical industry and orthodox medicine in the UK.

1 The cost to the nation of synthetic drugs, borne by the taxpayer, amounts to £2 billion annually.

2 Manufacturers of synthetic medicines spend approximately £50,000 per doctor in marketing their medicines.

3 The General Practitioner's knowledge of the drugs that he prescribes is generally considered to be unsatisfactory as their only source of information comes from the promotional literature of the drug companies themselves, which is invariably biased and incomplete.

4 Approximately 75% of all G.P. consultations end in the prescription of a pharmaceutical medicine though 40% of all patients never take their prescribed drugs.

5 It is estimated that drugs to the value of between £700-900 million are wasted each year through unnecessary prescribing and the reluctance of patients to take their prescribed medicines.

6 Iatrogenic illnesses (illness brought about by prescribed treatments) is widespread and accounts for between 15% and 40% of all illnesses. There are approximately 40,000 hospital admissions each year for overdoses of psychotropic drugs. One in ten geriatric admissions is believed to be as a result of iatrogenic illness.

7 Adverse drug reactions should be monitored by G.Ps but it is not in their interests to do this and incidences are therefore grossly under reported. The DHSS estimate that doctors only report about one in twenty of such adverse reactions.

8 Pharmaceutical medicines may be tested on laboratory animals but no one knows just what their side effects are until they are tested upon humans. There are about 4,000 deaths each year which are officially attributed to prescribed drugs. They are known as 'therapeutic misadventures'. However, it is generally agreed that the true figure is much higher. It is impossible to measure the influence of drug medicines as a causative factor of ill-health and as a contributory factor in death due

to the complexity of the body in its interaction with synthetic chemicals.

9 There have been a total of 2,000 fatalities officially linked with the drug Opren alone.

10 At this present time, herbal and natural medicines are under threat from government legislation which has demanded that alternative medicines be subjected to the same clinical trials as drug medicines. This is prohibitively expensive for small companies and may lead to many natural medicines disappearing. If a herbal medicine does not obtain a licence, though its use may date back throughout history, then no claim can be made for that medicine, making it unrecognisable and therefore unmarketable. It may not be surprising to learn that the *Committee for Review of Medicines* which makes all the decisions affecting the fate of herbal and alternative medicines, is comprised exclusively of doctors and members of the orthodox medical establishment. No representatives of alternative medicine have been invited onto the Committee. If you feel strongly about this matter and wish to preserve your freedom to choose herbal and natural medicines then join the *Natural Medicines Society* in their struggle, their address is at the back of the book, and lobby your MP.

Dr B W Halstead, an eminent American doctor, has this to say on the subject of modern medicine, 'There will be a medical edition of the Nuremberg Trials for the atrocities now being committed in the name of orthodox medicine; the needless loss of life, mutilation of bodies and imposition of excessive suffering, much of which is for the financial benefit of a ruthlessly powerful medical cartel, will not continue to be tolerated.'

Dr Robert Blomfield of St Stephen's Hospital, Chelsea, wrote in the Sunday Times, 'Most people buy what advertisers tell them to, and the doctors, who should be advising them, know no better. One has only to sample the average hospital meal to see how low on the list of priorities food comes in modern medicine. What is urgently needed is the widespread realisation that you are what you eat and drink and breathe and that if these factors deviate far from nature trouble and illness will ensue to a greater or lesser degree. If a fraction of the money spent on research into the treatment of disease was used to investigate the relationship of diet to disease, the health of people in this country could be dramatically improved across the board. But much of the research is financed by drug companies who have a vested interest, not surprisingly, in drug treatment. And if one looks at it closely, so have most doctors. Naturally grown, unprocessed foods are the basis of all good health, but amazingly this fundamental factor is almost, if not completely, neglected in British and American medical schools, where science rules the roost.'

Natural medicine recognises the need for a constitutional approach to disease treating the patient holistically on all levels, mind body and spirit, emphasising rehabilitation of the whole constitution through an observance of nature's laws. Treatment of any disease or condition of ill-health demands attention to the healing elements of nature as discussed in chapter. Diet is of particular importance in the prevention and treatment of disease and should comprise mainly plant foods such as fruits, vegetables, seeds, beans, nuts and cereal grains of wheat, oats, barley and brown rice with the inclusion of small quantities of animal foods as a compromise rather than a necessity preferring low fat dairy products to flesh foods. Where possible, food should be eaten raw as nature intended as this preserves its nutritional value, though some comprimise can be made in this matter as cooking does improve the palatability and flavour of some foods. It should be remembered, however, that man is the only animal that uses heat to cook food, an innovation for which he pays a heavy price in increased incidences of disease and ill-health. The need for cooked food is psychological in origin rather than physiological but again, a compromise can be made in this matter.

Nutritional and herbal remedies can be used for their therapeutic value in invigorating the bodys own healing powers, but these are largely beneficial only when combined with the eight healing forces. Treatment of any disease or ill health should always involve an all out effort to rebuild the constitution using the therapeutic forces of nature in their entirety. Even the correcting of a simple vitamin deficiency in the body is dependant upon an adequate diet furnishing all nutrients before the missing vitamin can be absorbed. All nutrients work synergistically in the body and are therefore interdependent and unable to operate in isolation. In the treatment of ill health all the healing forces should be observed with the adoption of a natural diet including nutritious foods such as brewers yeast, kelp, wheatgerm and molasses and whichever herbal or nutritious medicine specifically applies to a particular complaint. A return to the principles of natural medicine will not only confer good health on the individual but will make its contribution towards the protection of the environment.

Embracing vegetarianism or veganism will do much to alleviate the distress and pain of the animal kingdom and also will encourage the use of land for the growing of natural plant foods to feed the world's population rather than the inefficient conversion by cattle of plant foods into expensive animal proteins. The use of natural medicines and cosmetics will also spare the animal kingdom from the pain, suffering and indignity of cruel animal experiments. Scientific researchers defend such actions by maintaining that their work is for the benefit of humanity. Considering that natural cosmetics are as good if not better than those tested on animals and that health is maintained by pure food and the elements and not through blood letting, grotesque surgery, amputation and experimentation, the words of those involved in such research ring hollow indeed. When one considers man's brutality against man and his butchering and slaughtering of the animal kingdom, it is only to be hoped that the Law of Karma does indeed operate and that those responsible will be repaid their just deserts.

For every infringement against the laws of nature there is a price to be paid. If the occurrence of brain disease in cows can be brought about by the crass stupidity of feeding grass eating animals on sheep offal then the price that will have to be paid is likely to be the wholesale destruction of the planet. Whatever nature's reply, it is no more than man's treachery deserves. Hope for the future is yet possible but is confined to the development of man's consciousness and the flowering of higher sentiments of love, compassion and tolerance. How far the potential for consciousness and enlightenment is constrained by environmental or inherited factors is difficult to ascertain, but one can rest assured that compassion and tolerance towards one's fellow man and empathy towards nature is a pre-requisite to man's salvation from his own destructive greed and self interest. The rising tide of this consciousness at ground level, if not amongst those in power, should give some hope for the future and provide some degree of optimism and positivity in the midst of a troubled world.

In conclusion, it requires only to be restated that a diet of natural foods will play a large part in the maintaining and rebuilding health and vitality and reducing the ageing process to its natural pace. Mental attitude is an important factor in ageing as too many people in our society are conditioned into believing that they have reached old age, living out the part in appearance and behaviour, when such is not really the case. Remember that the Hunzas live up to the ripe old age of 140 years and 90 years of age is considered quite youthful.

If the principles of natural health are observed and allied with a substantial degree of positivity and mental dynamism, then vitality and well being can be maintained into a ripe old age. Positive thought in general can be a priceless asset in all walks of life due to its action in invigorating the neuro- endocrine system, making a positive contribution to the maintenance of good health. After all there are few benefits conferred upon the individual or the population in general from the deleterious and dispiriting consequences of negativity and negative emotion. Positive thought and its mastery is an area which offers boundless possibilities for the improvement of the quality of life and for the general well being and happiness of the individual. Alternatively, there is no question but that biochemical disharmony and enervation tend to induce negative emotion and the brutalisation of the spirit in which negative sentiments of intolerance, prejudice and ill feeling come to the forefront. The converse is also true that physical well being and biochemical harmony can induce a sense of positivity and of the joy of living and can predispose mankind towards higher sentiments of love, compassion and decency.

The pursuit of vitality and the liberation of the life force of the system would appear to be admirable goals, considering the enormous benefits conferred, of positivity, dynamism and improved quality of life. If a condition of vitality creates positivity then the converse is also true that low levels of vitality predisposes us towards negative feelings, whether of anxiety, self-doubt, depression or lowered self-esteem. It must be re-emphasised that nervous energy motivates every action and every thought and is the motive force of life itself. Nervous energy, as some might believe, is not liberated exclusively in times of stress and anxiety but is expended in all activities including physical work, mental thought and the digestion of food. It is possible to bankrupt the body's nervous energy in a variety of ways but it happens normally as a result of a combintation of factors occurring over a prolonged period of time including general overwork, poor diet, lack of fresh air and exercise, irregular work hours, particularly night work, lack of sleep and rest, abuse of alcohol and drugs and general unwholesome habits of living combined with a degree of self neglect. The discrepancy between a natural lifestyle as might occur in the land of Hunza with its natural preservation of vitality, and that of an individual caught up in twentieth century Britain should illuminate the reasons for the inevitable ill-health and loss of vitality witnessed in our society.

Furthermore, it seems highly likely that due to the increasingly complex and taxing nature of modern society and to the politics of age with its promotion of self-interest and the 'survival of the fittest' mentality, stress and overwork will feature more prominently throughout the nineties with the inevitable consequence of a dramatic escalation in the number of people suffering from dissipation of their vital force and nervous exhaustion. Those who exhaust their life force or nervous energy to a marked degree can descend into an abyss of suffering which is a vision of Hell itself. Clearly there are degrees of severity of nerve exhaustion but it is to be strongly recommended that early warning signs be recognised and heeded, and the healing force of nature implemented to effect recovery.

The preservation and development of nervous energy and vitality can clearly be seen as an important prerequisite to the full enjoyment of life, to the ability to cope with the stresses and strains of the modern world and to the preservation of emotional health and wellbeing. In the quest for happiness, a pursuit in which we all take part, the acquisition of vitality and physical health, maintained by a healthy lifestyle and a diet of natural foods would appear to be the first step for those who wish to assume responsibility for the quality of their own lives.

From whatever angle and on whatever time scale one considers the human condition or the nature of man's existence on planet earth, (excluding the obvious purpose or destination), it would appear that the gift of life which has been bestowed on us should be cherished and enjoyed for the unique experience that it is. Should this planet destroy itself in an explosion of greed and self-interest, then it will be of no great consequence to the surrounding universe, the only loss will be ours. In the constant struggle between good and evil in which we find ourselves embroiled, it is only possible to remain positive in the face of adversity until such a time as human consciousness aspires to a level of greater feeling, compassion and empathy. It is quite unfortunate that world leaders, whether elected or self-appointed, tend to lack true qualities of compassion and humanity which are so invaluable to the future of this planet and to the human condition. We should also be on guard against misinformation presented by those in power and authority who wish only to maintain their own privileged positions and vested interests.

Attacks by conventional medicine on alternative therapies has become more vehement since natural treatments have become more popular. This outrageous scenario is likely to be re-enacted repeatedly in the future with those with the most to lose being the most outspoken in their criticism. The Imperial Cancer Research Fund recently conducted research into the effectiveness of holistic therapies carried out at the Bristol Cancer help Centre, finding their methods ineffective. The Imperial Cancer Research Fund collects millions of pounds in charity annually and yet preoccupies itself with the search for a pharmaceutical solution to cancer without showing any inclination towards researching the dietary and environmental causes of cancer. The reason for this must be left to their own conscience.

Through observance of the physical laws of nature and the liberation of positive thought and dynanism and a degree of faith in the innate goodness of man and the possibilities which abound in the development of man's consciousness, it ought to be possible to improve to a greater extent the quality of one's life. Some perserverance and determination will be required initially in the adoption of a natural lifestyle and a diet of natural foods, but it should be seen as a glorious challenge which can be undertaken with enthusiasm and anticipation.

Books on vegetarianism and veganism abound in libraries and bookshops and the challenge to make delicious wholesome meals from natural foods should inspire the individual to undreamed of artistic heights! However, while the pursuit of health and vitality may be valuable goals, they should not be goals in themselves but prerequisites to the greater end of happiness and the enjoyment of life itself. There would appear to be little value in living out a life of abject boredom and misery through obsessive obedience to nature's laws. Nature allows some leeway in the observance of her decrees and is well able to make concessions to the social enjoyment of life and to the pursuit of pleasure, particularly if the main principles of health are observed.

Besides, happiness itself should be the main goal in life with health and vitality subservient to this end. Neither should happiness nor the enjoyment of life be overlooked as important factors in the maintenance of good health.

Mixing socially can be one of life's most fulfilling and rewarding pleasures and if combined with strictly moderate intakes of alcohol, then the benefits can outweigh the disadvantages. Alcohol is much abused in our society, creating ill-health and unhappiness but if consumed in small quantities it does appear to be of some therapeutic value. Besides, in a violent nuclear age and in consideration of the arduous and fickle nature of life it may not be wise to postpone or forego too many of life's pleasures for too long, though moderation and emotional poise have much to recommend them.

Furthermore, it is not intended that harmony with nature should confer sainthood on the individual. On the contrary, through increased vitality and well-being, it should be possible to approach the enjoyment of life with greater dynamism and enthusiasm, all the better able to tolerate life's less than wholesome but nevertheless enjoyable forms of pleasure!

BIBLIOGRAPHY

Everybody's Guide to nature Cure, Harry Benjamin,
Health For All Publishing Co 1976

Lets Get Well, Adelle Davis, Unwin paperbacks 1966

Lets Stay Healthy, Adelle Davis, Unwin paperbacks 1982

Potter New Cyclopaedia of Botanical Drugs and Preparations, R C Wren,
Health Science Press 1907

The Encyclopaedia of Natural Health, Max Warmbrand, Souvenir press 1962

Food for a Future, Jon Wynne-Tyson, Centaur Press 1975

The Sunfood Way to Health, Dugald Semple, Health For All 1956

Culpeppers Colour Herbal, Nicholas Culpepper, W Foulsham & Co Ltd 1983

Feverfew, Dr Stewart Johnson, Sheldon Press 1984

Feverfew, Britt and Kean, Century 1987

Candida Albicans, Leon Chaitow, Thorsons 1985

Arthritis, Cause and Control, Dr Barton Wright, Bunterbird Ltd

Arthritis Self Help, Leon Chaitow, Thorsons 1987

A Doctors Proven New Home Cure for Arthitis, Girand Campbell, Thorsons 1979

Arthritis the Conquest, Harry Clements, Thorsons 1968

Evening Primrose Oil, Judy Graham, Thorsons 1984

The Eight Week Cholesterol Cure, Kowalski, Thorsons 1987

The Bristol Diet, Dr Alec Forbes, Century Arrow 1984

The Bristol Programme, Penny Brohn Century Paperbacks 1987

Cancer: The Alternative Method of Treatment, Dr Isaac Bryant,
Roberts Publications 1983

Cancer: How to prevent it, G E Berkley, Spectrum 1978

Killing Cancer, Jason Winters, Vinton Publishing 1980

Cancer: Its Dietetic Cause and Cure, Dr Maud Tresillian Fere, Gateway Book Co 1963

A Gentle Way with Cancer, Brenda Kidman, Century Arrow 1983

Thorsons Complete Guide to Vitamins and Minerals, Leonard Mervyn, Thorsons 1986

The Vitamin Bible, Earl Mindell, Artington Books 1979